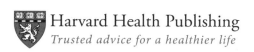
Harvard Health Publishing
Trusted advice for a healthier life

Dear Reader,

Health information generally centers on avoiding or treating diseases, such as heart disease or cancer. But if you look at what characterizes good health as you age, it's not just sidestepping illnesses like these; it's whether you are strong and capable. Can you move easily and without pain? Can you remain independent and self-sufficient? Can you stay in your home, or will you need to move to assisted living or a nursing home? In short, can you stay "in the game"?

These are issues that concern everyone. Problems with mobility—such as slowed walking or difficulty rising out of a chair—are often the first signs of a decline in health and day-to-day function. That's why the medical community has put a growing focus on helping people maintain mobility and safeguard independence as they age.

Some of that work should ideally begin decades before you begin to experience mobility issues. Many of the health problems that come with aging could be avoided or lessened by adopting practices like exercising, building muscle strength, following a balanced diet, and maintaining a healthy weight in your 40s and 50s. But even at older ages—and even if you are already facing declining health or a loss of independence—simple steps toward better health and physical conditioning can improve your abilities and help prevent further loss of movement.

The goal of this Special Health Report is to help you achieve this. It will show you how mobility relies on many body systems working together: your bones, muscles, and joints; your senses, brain, and balance system. It will help you understand common age-related changes and health conditions that cause people to begin losing their ability to move. It translates clinical and scientific knowledge about mobility into practical steps you can take to stay healthy and strong.

As you will see, this report will encourage you to challenge your body with regular physical activity and exercises that have been shown to preserve or improve mobility. But mobility is measured not just by the flights of stairs you can climb, but also by your confidence in executing daily tasks, your willingness to keep moving, and your effort to maintain connections to loved ones and to the wider world. In addition, when mobility starts to present a challenge, you need to be open to high-tech solutions, assistive devices, and services that give you the support you need to remain independent.

Whatever your age or health status, now is the time to ensure an active and capable future.

Sincerely,

Scott D. Martin, M.D.
Medical Editor

Harvard Health Publishing | Harvard Medical School | 4 Blackfan Circle, 4th Floor | Boston, MA 02115

Mobility and quality of life

When you're young and healthy, you never stop to consider how marvelous it is to be able to move effortlessly. You get out of bed in the morning, take a shower, then head downstairs to your kitchen to make coffee. You begin the day's activities, whatever those may entail. You think nothing of driving across town to meet a good friend for lunch. On the way home, maybe you go to the grocery store to pick up a few things for dinner, then carry the bags to the car and drive home.

Even the simple, relatively uneventful day described here requires a great deal of physical stamina, strength, balance, coordination, and range of motion. It requires the ability to get out of bed easily, take a shower, manage a flight of stairs, walk a quarter- or half-mile easily, get in and out of a car, navigate traffic, and carry bags. Most of us spend our lives doing these tasks day in and day out without marveling at how much our bodies can do. But when we lose these basic skills because of a health problem or the physical decline associated with aging, we begin to understand how much living well relies on being able to move.

Mobility problems are common. Statistics from the CDC indicate that close to 14% of American adults have a mobility issue that profoundly affects their ability to walk and climb stairs. Balance issues also tend to occur, along with gait changes over time.

Maybe you're relatively young, and joint replacement surgery or physical therapy for an injury is all you need to get back on your feet. This report will address issues like those. It will also address the deeper, more entrenched mobility problems that come with older age, because, increasingly, there are effective ways of coping—whether with canes and high-tech wheelchairs or with a wide variety of services that can help keep you living on your own.

In addition, this report will look at things you should be doing at every stage of life to promote your health, because ultimately, those, too, play a role in how well you age and therefore how mobile you remain. These include measures such as the following:

- maintaining muscle strength and power
- taking care of the joints you need for walking
- caring for your back and posture
- building your sense of balance, to avoid falls
- strengthening core muscles for better stability
- protecting your eyes and ears, and keeping your brain sharp
- maintaining a healthy weight
- ensuring that your home and environment help rather than hinder your mobility.

These measures can all add up to a healthier future—and greater mobility and independence.

The importance of mobility

Mobility is defined as your ability to move purposefully around your environment. At first, an impairment might not seem like a big deal—you learn to move more slowly and deliberately, or you work around the problem by relying on a cane or walker. But this can

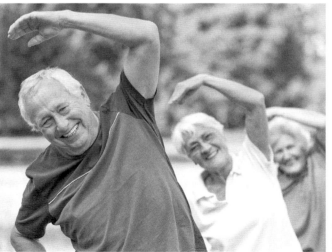

To maintain the ability to walk, it's important to stay active—or, if you haven't been active for a while, to start with whatever simple measures it takes to boost your level of physical activity.

lead to a spiral of poor health. As you move less, you may gain weight, stop exercising, and withdraw from social relationships and activities that stimulate you mentally. Not exercising can make many health conditions worse. The resulting physical, emotional, and mental decline further restricts your mobility.

Mobility problems are linked with lower quality of life and higher rates of depression. Over time, these limitations raise your risk of becoming disabled—unable to perform daily activities because of a physical or mental impairment. That's why it's important to intervene to either prevent future mobility impairments or reduce existing ones.

Most importantly, mobility issues can lead to a loss of independence and can make it impossible for you to live on your own. Even if technology allows you to overcome some challenges, for most people, the ability to rely on their own bodies, skills, and mental agility is a crucial part of living a satisfying life. The vast majority of people would rather have the capacity to do all the simple acts described earlier than depend on caretakers and assistive devices.

Measuring mobility

Do you have trouble walking a quarter of a mile? Can you climb stairs on your own and accomplish basic daily tasks like cooking, showering, and going to the grocery store? These are the kinds of questions that clinicians ask when trying to assess mobility limitations. Here are some other factors a doctor, nurse, or physical therapist might use to assess mobility in patients who exhibit a potential mobility problem, because of either an injury (from an accident or a fall, for example) or a chronic condition like arthritis.

Gait. Human walking requires a series of movements: lifting the foot, placing it on the ground ahead of you, and shifting your weight from the heel to the ball of the foot. The way you walk is called your gait. Changes in the speed or pattern of your gait can give your doctor an indication of mobility trouble.

People's gait often changes with age: healthy people in their 70s generally have a 10% to 20% reduction in the speed and the length of their stride compared with healthy people in their 20s. A more cautious, shuffling,

wider-base gait may be the result of compensating for problems with vision and hearing or with bones and muscles. Arthritis often makes people adopt a flat-footed gait or may result in a bent posture that significantly alters walking patterns as the body's center of gravity shifts forward. Chronic pain and a host of medical conditions can also cause gait abnormalities. Over time, gait changes can weaken or cause an imbalance in the muscles you use to walk, compounding health problems and predisposing you to falls.

To assess your gait, a doctor or physical therapist might have you walk about 10 feet across a room while timing you; managing the walk relatively quickly is a sign of good health. An uneven, halting, or shuffling gait is often a sign of an underlying health problem.

The "timed up and go" (TUG) test. In another common test, you sit in a chair, and when prompted, rise up and walk about 10 feet in a line, then turn and come back to the chair and sit down. Most people with normal mobility can complete the task in less than 12 seconds. If you take 12 seconds or longer, it indicates an increased risk for falling. How you accomplish the TUG test—for example, whether you shuffle or have to steady yourself or don't swing your arms while walking—can also indicate if you have muscle weakness, posture or balance problems, or joint pain.

Simple tasks. A mobility assessment will also focus on how you handle simple tasks and challenges, like stepping over objects on the floor, balancing on one leg, balancing on both feet positioned one in front of the other, and rising from a chair and sitting down several times in a row.

Daily activities. One of the best clues to your mobility is how well you accomplish small daily tasks like bathing, preparing meals, cleaning the house, and going shopping. Many people who have trouble moving still do these tasks, but they may change the way they do them—sitting on a chair in the shower, for instance.

Range of travel. There's a difference between what people *can* do and what they actually do. Mobility researchers have developed tools like the Life-Space Assessment, which looks at how much people travel in their daily routines (for example, leaving the house, visiting places in their neighborhoods, or going to other communities) as a way of representing their actual mobility in daily life. The advantage of such a tool is that it takes into account real-world adaptations you use to boost your mobility (for example, using a cane or wheelchair, driving, or using public transportation) as well as nonphysical factors that affect mobility (such as depression, lack of motivation, or lack of financial resources).

Improving your mobility

People often deny or ignore changes in their gait or their ability to perform routine tasks and are hesitant to bring these issues up with their doctors. Instead, they may try to adapt and narrow down their lives to manage the changes and prevent falls. But treatment can make a big difference in outcomes. For example, doctors can prescribe balance and gait-training exercises if changes are caught early in the process.

A fundamental goal of healthy aging is to keep walking as long as possible. Of course, people who lose their ability to walk can still retain mobility through wheelchairs and other assistive devices, and they can have full and happy lives. But there's no reason why most people can't keep walking their whole lives. To maintain this ability, it's important to stay active—or, if you haven't been active for a while, to start with whatever measures it takes to boost your level of activity.

It can't be emphasized enough: engaging in physical activity is the single most important thing you can do to maintain mobility and independence, no matter your age or your health status. It can help you control your weight. It's the key to keeping your muscles and bones strong, your joints working properly, your heart healthy, and your metabolism revved. The more you move, the better your strength and balance will be, and the less likely you will be to fall or lose the ability to perform basic daily functions. And that's on top of all the other health benefits of regular exercise, such as reduced risks of cardiovascular disease, type 2 diabetes, and some cancers. Exercise even has positive effects on mood and may help improve cognitive function.

In addition to doing targeted exercises for muscle strength and flexibility, joint health, and balance as described in this report, you should strive to increase routine daily physical activities that aren't formal exercise, such as climbing stairs. If you're in pain, all this activity may seem impossible. But in many cases, exercise actually helps reduce the pain. If you have osteoarthritis, for example, regular exercise not only helps maintain joint function, but also relieves stiffness and diminishes pain and fatigue. Maintaining muscle strength can also help dampen stresses on joints.

How much exercise do you need? For healthy adults, the Physical Activity Guidelines for Americans from the U.S. Department of Health and Human Services recommend 150 to 300 minutes of moderate exercise a week, with activity every day. The guidelines also recommend twice-weekly strength training sessions and balance exercises for older adults at risk of falling. Disability should not be a reason to refrain from all activity. The guidelines state: "When older adults cannot do 150 minutes of moderate-intensity aerobic activity a week because of chronic conditions, they should be as physically active as their abilities and conditions allow." Even modest efforts count. "Move more and sit less throughout the day," the guidelines advise. "Some activity is better than none."

The key is finding activities you can do and enjoy. If your joints are the problem, don't try to "pace" your joints—let your joints pace you. For example, don't make yourself go jogging. Instead, pick low-impact activities, such as swimming or water aerobics. Try cycling on a stationary bike at the gym or at home. Yoga, tai chi, and qigong are other good alternatives. Even a gentle walking program that ramps up slowly will help. In other words, there's a lot of flexibility in the kinds of activities you do and when. Don't feel guilty if you can't do the same kinds of activities you used to. The important thing is not to let joint pain keep you from being physically active.

If you're in doubt about your ability to take on even a modest exercise program, we recommend filling out the Get Active Questionnaire (GAQ), a tool developed by the Canadian Society for Exercise Physiology to help people determine whether they should talk to a doctor before embarking on, or ramping up, an exercise program. You can find it at www.health. harvard.edu/GAQ. Whether or not you use the GAQ, we recommend talking to a doctor about whether it's safe to exercise if any of the following applies:

- You've had hip or knee surgery.
- You've been experiencing pain in your hip, knee, foot and ankle, or back.
- You have a chronic or unstable health condition, such as heart disease, or you have a respiratory ailment, high blood pressure, osteoporosis, diabetes, or several risk factors for heart disease.

Mind, mood, and mobility

Most mobility tests measure what your body is capable of doing. But your mind is just as important in determining how much you move in your daily life. Often, a health setback like a fall or arthritis pain saps people's confidence or their willingness to venture outside the house. You may give up driving or stop taking walks. Eventually, you mostly stay home, and your movements become slower, stiffer, and more halting. This loss of mobility can further worsen health problems. It can also diminish your connections with friends and loved ones and your engagement in activities you enjoy. It can affect your mood, leading to depression. You might stop following a daily schedule and fall into poor dietary habits, either gaining weight that further hinders movement, or eating too little and losing energy and resilience.

This cycle of reduced mobility, poor psychological health, and physical deterioration can stem from a life change—such as the death of a spouse—as much as from a health problem. Your mind, mood, and mobility are intrinsically linked. That's why maintaining your emotional health and mental engagement are so important for healthy aging.

If your actual mobility does not match your physical capabilities, it's important to ask why. Is depression, loneliness, anxiety, or fear slowing you down? Are you struggling with retirement or the death of a loved one? Consider talking about these issues with your doctor, a mental health professional, or a trusted friend. Think about what motivates you to move— what are your reasons to get up in the morning? It might be family, social connections, volunteer work, shopping, cultural experiences, enjoying nature, or walking a dog. Build more of these motivating experiences into your life to maintain your emotional and physical health. Establish some daily and weekly routines; following a schedule helps you stay active even when your mood or motivation flags.

Seeing a geriatrician

It's not unusual to see the same doctor for decades. But in old age, it's wise to consider switching to a geriatrician or at least consulting one. Geriatricians have expertise in dealing with many chronic conditions that are common in older adults—such as heart ailments, high blood pressure, diabetes, and disabilities. They are trained to consider the needs of the whole person and focus on function and quality of life. Some geriatricians routinely make home visits to see how you live and what changes could improve safety, nutrition, function, and mobility. Usually, they recognize the importance of allowing family members to attend appointments.

Geriatricians are also well aware of the harmful effects that medications can have on older people. It's common for older people to take multiple medications, because they often have numerous health problems. The more medications you take, the higher the risk of drug interactions and harmful side effects, such as increased risk of falls. Older people are especially vulnerable because of age-related changes in body composition: since you have less muscle mass, your body processes drugs differently than younger people's do. Even over-the-counter medications can contribute to this problem, and the effects can be cumulative. A review of 14 studies found that each year, about 11% of older adults experience adverse drug events, and 10% of those reactions require a hospital stay.

A comprehensive geriatric evaluation can offer wide-ranging advice that vastly improves your quality of life and ability to live independently. That might include recommendations to change or discard medications, consult with a physical therapist or occupational therapist, adapt your home, pursue neuropsychological testing, or add home care services. Medicare or Medicaid will pay for the evaluation. Some private insurance plans also provide coverage if the primary care physician makes a referral. ◗

Prime movers: Knees and hips

Mobility relies on the body's two largest joints, the hips and knees. You ask a lot of both these joints: they must bear your full weight and coordinate movement over a lifetime of standing, walking, running, dancing, and sports. Not surprisingly, hip and knee pain are common complaints, and nearly everyone who lives into old age can expect some pain or loss of function in these joints.

For people with severe pain, joint replacements and other medical advances have dramatically improved mobility. Advances in our understanding of how to care for the joints—through better preventive exercise and rehabilitation—have also helped many people regain mobility they had lost or recover from surgery more quickly. Taking care of your hips and knees and managing pain so that it doesn't slow you down will help you avoid losing mobility as you age.

How knees and hips work

Both hips and knees are critical load-bearing joints. The knee is where three bones come together: the femur (thighbone), tibia (shin bone), and patella (kneecap). The simplest way to think about the knee is as a hinge in one plane, like the lid on a box. But in fact, the joint is more complicated than a simple hinge, allowing greater movement; every time you flex or extend the knee, there is a small amount of rotation, sliding, and rolling of the bones to keep them properly aligned. Muscles around the knee keep this complex movement stable.

The hip, too, is a complicated joint. It involves bones, muscles, and other tissues extending beyond the hip bone to the upper thigh, groin, and buttocks. The joint itself has a ball-and-socket structure with a wide range of motion, so it's capable of more types of movement than the knee, like swinging the legs to the side or rotating them out so you can sit cross-legged. But all of this mobility, combined with the need to support your body weight, makes the hip susceptible to injury, pain, and loss of mobility if any of its components aren't working correctly.

General knee and hip care

Good self-care of your joints is important. Here are some rules to follow when you have an injury, osteoarthritis, or any other health condition that affects your ankles, knees, and also the hips to some extent.

RICE for injuries

RICE—rest, ice, compression, and elevation—is a first-aid strategy for most musculoskeletal injuries, including those involving the knees and hips. For knees, it is sometimes the only treatment you need.

Rest doesn't necessarily mean lying in bed or on the couch—in fact, inactivity can make injuries worse by causing stiffness around the joints and weakening the muscles. Instead, rest means avoiding the type of

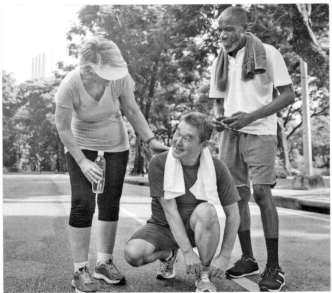

You ask a lot of your hips and knees. They must bear your full weight and coordinate movement over a lifetime of standing, walking, running, dancing, and sports.

activity that directly led to the injury, and trying low-impact activities that keep pressure off the joint.

Ice can reduce swelling by shrinking injured blood vessels, and it also eases pain. Use a homemade or store-bought ice pack, and apply it to the injured area for 20 minutes at a time, with 20-minute pauses in between. (Note: Never apply ice directly to skin, but rather make sure you put a layer of cloth or other material between the ice and your skin to protect you from frostbite.) Devices are also available that apply continuous cold to joints by using circulating cold water rather than ice, but these should also be used with 20-minute breaks between cooling sessions. Ice helps knee injuries of all types. For hip injuries deep in the joint, ice isn't effective because the cold can't penetrate that far, but it can still help with hip pain stemming from problems closer to the surface.

Compression can promote recovery by reducing swelling and providing support to the knee or ankle after an injury. Wearing a stretchy neoprene support or wrapping an elastic bandage around an injured knee or ankle provides compression, but take care that the wrap isn't so tight that the skin below the joint becomes cool or blue.

Elevation—raising an injured leg and propping it on a pillow or stool—can also reduce swelling by preventing blood from pooling at the site of the injury.

Heat for long-term pain and stiffness

Icing is the best therapy in the first day or two after an injury because it reduces swelling; after that, applying heat can help ease pain. Heat reduces discomfort by relieving stiffness and promoting flexibility in the muscles. Some people like to use heat in the morning and before exercising or stretching, and ice after a workout or at the end of the day. You can use a store-bought heating pad, or heat a damp towel in the microwave for 20-second increments until it reaches the desired temperature. Make sure the heat you're applying feels warm, not hot, to avoid burning the skin, and don't leave it on for more than 20 minutes. A warm bath is a mainstay of physical therapy for joints and muscles. You don't need a professional whirlpool bath to get the benefits; soaking in a hot bath or hot tub or even taking a hot shower can work as well.

Physical therapy and exercise

While you may need to rest your joints after injuries, exercise is also an important part of recovering from an injury or managing a health condition like osteoarthritis. Often the first treatments for joint pain will be an over-the-counter pain medication combined with physical therapy or a set of specific exercises.

A physical therapist often works with an orthopedist to help you carry out a program of movements to treat your specific condition. Physical therapy typically involves one or more sessions of supervised exercises combined with exercises that you do regularly at home. The primary goal is often to increase the range of motion in a joint, using stretches and movements that gently take a joint to the edge of its range. Another goal is to strengthen specific muscles around a joint, which can correct some joint-related problems or provide better support to dampen the stresses on knees and hips. Balance exercises (see page 34) can also help you keep joints stable and avoid injuries.

Mobility aids

Canes and walkers are simple tools, but they've been shown to improve stability, prevent falls, and take a load off painful hips or knees. If you're recovering from an injury or surgery, struggling with arthritis, or managing a balance impairment, a cane or walker can help you stay active and avoid further disability (see "Mobility devices: Choosing a cane or walker," page 8). Still, many people feel reluctant or embarrassed to use them. If your doctor recommends one, don't let your sense of pride keep you from using it. Whatever weight you place on a cane is weight taken off your hip or knee. These devices should be part of a larger plan for your mobility, which may include muscle-strengthening exercises, a treatment plan for a condition, and regular walks and physical activity.

How osteoarthritis slows you down

One of the most common causes of impaired mobility is osteoarthritis, which affects 32.5 million Americans. This condition causes a breakdown of the cartilage that wraps over the ends of bones (known medically as articular cartilage) and sometimes affects surround-

Mobility devices: Choosing a cane or walker

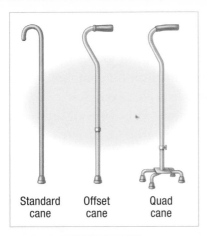

Standard cane   Offset cane   Quad cane

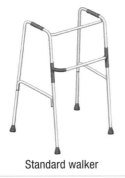

Standard walker

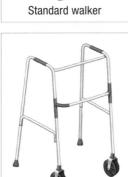

Two-wheel walker

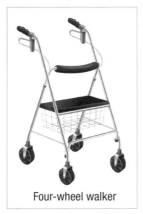

Four-wheel walker

If you have mobility issues or you've just gone through surgery, a cane or walker can be the key to maintaining your independence and staying active. These tools will help keep you on your feet and prevent falls.

Canes and walkers come in a few different varieties. Your physical therapist can tell you which type is most appropriate for your needs. Here's a quick guide:

Standard canes typically come in wood or aluminum, with a curved or T-shaped handle. They're reasonably priced and lightweight, and some fold for easier storage. A standard cane will improve your base of support, but it won't bear a lot of weight.

Offset canes have a handle that curves away from and then toward you. They're designed to support more weight than a standard cane, and they may be helpful if you have painful arthritis in your hip or knee.

Quad canes have four legs. They provide more support and can bear more weight than a standard or offset cane. But because you'll need to plant all four legs firmly on the ground for stability, this type of cane can slow you down.

Standard walkers have four rubber-tipped legs. This is the most stable type of walker, but you'll need to pick it up and put it down with each step in order to move.

Two-wheel walkers have two wheels in the front and two rubber-tipped legs in the back. They move along more easily than a standard walker, while still offering a good amount of stability.

Four-wheel walkers (rollators) enable you to move quickly, but you can't put as much weight on them as you can with a standard or two-wheel walker.

ing tissues as well (see Figure 1, page 9). With less protective cushioning between the bones, the normally frictionless motion of the joint becomes difficult. The result is pain, swelling, stiffness, and less ability to move. If the cartilage continues to break down over time, the bones may begin to rub together, which can permanently damage the joint.

Osteoarthritis can occur in any joint, but the knees and hips are common sites because of the weight they bear. The hands are also often affected. Osteoarthritis develops over time, and there is no known cure. The best way to prevent it is to avoid gaining excess weight, to strive for a healthy weight if you're overweight, and to stay active while avoiding injuries that can happen when you exercise improperly or put too much stress on the joints.

Osteoarthritis can make it difficult to accomplish activities you once managed easily. Compensating for the diseased joints can leave muscles tired. While the pain might improve early in the day as you move around, many people find the pain gets worse later in the day as their muscles grow fatigued, leaving them more sensitive to joint stress. Osteoarthritis and other health conditions that cause chronic pain often limit movement psychologically as well as physically. People may begin to associate activity and exercise with pain, and avoid opportunities to get out and move. That's why seeking treatment for osteoarthritis can help you preserve mobility; managing the symptoms helps you stay active with less pain. As the disease progresses, you and your doctor can discuss whether surgery and joint replacement may be good options.

The incidence of osteoarthritis is rising, and the disease is striking people earlier in life. Genetic predisposition can play a role in its development, and women are more likely to have it than men. But neither one explains why the caseload is rising or why osteoarthritis of the knees and hips is striking younger people. The increase in overweight and obesity in the United States may be one reason. Another likely factor is sports-related injuries and strain from exercise or overuse of joints. Competitive sports and other intense activities that put pressure on joints, such as long-distance running, soccer, or weight lifting, can increase the risk of developing osteoarthritis. So paradoxically, either a sedentary lifestyle or one filled with extreme activities can wind up causing problems that eventually affect mobility.

Treating osteoarthritis

If you do develop arthritis, managing it well can help keep you mobile. There is currently no proven way to reverse the damage. But treatments can help protect the joint from further injury, relieve symptoms, and keep you as active as possible. Treatments for osteoarthritis include the following:

Weight loss. Although it's not clear whether losing excess weight can prevent arthritis from getting worse, it can reduce symptoms by lightening the load on joints. With each step on level ground, you put one to one-and-a-half times your body weight on one knee. For a 200-pound person, that's up to 300 pounds of pressure on the knee. Off level ground, the news is worse: each knee bears two to three times your body weight when you go up and down stairs, and four to five times your body weight when you squat to tie a shoelace or pick up an item you dropped.

Physical therapy and exercise. You may need to rest your joints when pain flares up, but for the most part it's important to keep exercising in order to maintain your mobility, while avoiding high-impact activities like running and jumping that make symptoms worse (see "Staying active with joint pain," page 10). For knee osteoarthritis, physical therapists can help you practice movements that strengthen the muscles around your knee and maintain flexibility in the joint. If you have osteoarthritis of the hip, they can show you exercises to improve the hip's range of motion and promote strength and flexibility of the surrounding muscles in the hip, back, and pelvis. They can also help with strategies for accomplishing daily tasks and activities with less pain.

Ice or heat. Ice can reduce inflammation and ease pain, while heat can both ease pain and reduce stiffness. You can use either or both for osteoarthritis depending on what works best for you. Just be sure not to fall asleep with an ice or heat pack on your body or you could develop permanent burn marks on the skin. Apply the pack for 20 minutes, remove it for 20 minutes, and reapply it for another 20 minutes if you need further relief (see "Heat for long-term pain and stiffness," page 7).

Pain relief medications. Doctors can prescribe treatments to relieve pain and inflammation, so you can accomplish daily tasks more easily. Often, pain relief focuses on using one or more over-the-counter pain relievers such as acetaminophen (Tylenol), nonsteroidal anti-inflammatory drugs (NSAIDs) like ibuprofen (Advil) and naproxen (Aleve), or the topical NSAID gel diclofenac (Voltaren Arthritis Pain). It's best to limit use of these medications to two weeks at a time, unless otherwise directed by your doctor.

Wraps, braces, and orthotics. For early, mild knee arthritis with sudden flare-ups, a simple wrap or sleeve made of neoprene or elastic may help relieve pain. Because the sleeve itself doesn't provide much support to the joint, any benefit is thought to come

---

Figure 1: Joint changes in osteoarthritis

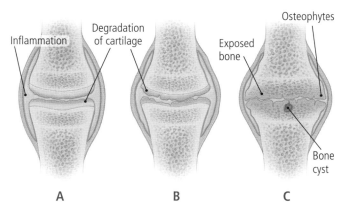

A. The first signs of osteoarthritis are microscopic pits and fissures on the cartilage surface, which are sometimes accompanied by inflammation.

B. The contours of the joint change, and the cartilage thins.

C. The bone surface thickens, and osteophytes (abnormal bony growths) develop over time. Cartilage continues to wear away. The joint space narrows until it nearly disappears, leaving bone rubbing against bone. In some arthritic knees, bone cysts (open spaces filled with fluid) can develop as a reaction to stress on the bone.

from improvements in the knee's position and movement. A physical therapist may prescribe a variation on this type of wrap that incorporates pulsed electrical stimulation, which has proved especially effective in treating knee osteoarthritis.

Various types of braces may also help. For example, if you have arthritis affecting only one part of the knee joint, a type of brace known as an unloader brace may help by taking some of the pressure off that part of the knee and redistributing the weight. Orthotic shoe inserts may also help people with knee arthritis, because flat feet and other foot problems can affect the alignment of the ankle and knee, placing additional stress on the joints. You can also take pressure off the knee with a cane or with a walking stick from an outdoor recreation store.

Injections. Injecting a long-acting corticosteroid drug into the knee or hip joint can ease pain temporarily. But most doctors recommend using this treatment sparingly—just two to three times per year—because it can damage joints when used too often. Injections of hyaluronic acid, a lubricating fluid normally found in joints, are sometimes given to people who don't experience relief from pain medications. Platelet-rich plasma (PRP) is also now being injected into arthritic joints, although there is little evidence on how well it works to relieve arthritis pain. PRP injections are also expensive, and insurance does not cover them.

Cooled radiofrequency ablation (Coolief). If medications and injections aren't working—and you don't want joint replacement surgery or aren't a good candidate for it—cooled radiofrequency ablation (called Coolief) is an option. It isn't a cure for osteoarthritis: it doesn't correct the underlying problems with your bones or cartilage or stop the progression of the disease. But it does reduce your pain by ablating (killing) the sensory nerves around the knee.

This minimally invasive, nonsurgical procedure is performed under local anesthesia in ambulatory surgical suites. It delivers radiofrequency energy via the tip of a probe, which is inserted into the region of sensory nerves around the knee. The doctor targets the pain-causing nerves, heating them with enough energy from the probe to ablate them. The device is cooled by water, which allows a larger area to be treated without danger of overheating the surrounding tissue. The procedure typically needs to be repeated every six to 12 months, since the nerves tend to regenerate. But recovery is quick—you can usually walk after the procedure. A review of 17 studies found radiofrequency ablation reduced pain for up to a year with few side effects.

Surgery. Many people ultimately require joint replacement surgery for arthritic knees and hips (see "Joint replacement," page 11). For most people, surgery is a second line of defense, used only after more conservative treatments fail or if the arthritis has progressed to a point where it is interfering with your mobility or has the potential to lead to permanent damage. In some cases, a doctor may recommend another surgical option besides replacement. For example:

- **Realignment (osteotomy) of the knee** is a procedure in which a surgeon reshapes the tibia and femur to improve the knee's alignment. It is often recommended for people with limited damage to the knee and those who are young, still highly active, or overweight.

- **Hip resurfacing** may offer an attractive alternative to traditional hip replacement, but only for a small segment of the population. The surgeon reshapes the head of the thighbone (instead of removing it as in total hip replacement) and caps it with a cobalt-chromium prosthetic that fits into a metal lining in the socket. The FDA has imposed a moratorium on the procedure for most people because rubbing of metal against metal can cause particles of cobalt

Staying active with joint pain

It's important to keep joints moving, even if you're dealing with pain from arthritis or an overuse injury. Sometimes you'll need to keep weight off a painful joint, but don't let that prevent you from exercising altogether. Set realistic goals, and if your overall health allows it, try these joint-friendly options:

- elliptical trainer
- stationary bike (recumbent or upright)
- tai chi
- swimming, water aerobics, or water walking
- rowing machine
- short walks throughout the day, instead of a long walk.

and chromium to come loose. This can lead to an autoimmune response that damages bone and tissue around the hip joint. Currently, hip resurfacing can only be performed in this country in young, active men who have end-stage arthritis. It is still popular in Europe.

- **Cartilage replacement (chondrocyte grafting)** involves grafting new cartilage tissue into pockets of damaged knee cartilage. Cartilage cells can be grown in a lab from a sample from the patient's own cartilage or from a donor and then transplanted into the diseased joint. This technique appears to be most helpful for people with less severe defects in cartilage.

- **Arthroscopic surgery,** which is done with tiny instruments through small incisions, may be used in a joint to remove torn cartilage, debris, and loose material. Although this approach has been used to treat osteoarthritis of the knee, multiple studies have questioned its usefulness for most arthritis cases. It is more helpful in people who have a tear in a meniscus from a sudden injury or a large piece of cartilage floating in the joint space. (A meniscus is a cartilage pad that provides cushioning in the knee joint.)

Joint replacement

Joint replacement is one of the most common elective surgeries in the United States, with more than one million procedures performed annually. Doctors recommend joint replacement in cases of severe osteoarthritis in which the joint shows significant deterioration. Because severe disease in the knee or hip can impede mobility and joint function, this surgery is most often recommended for those particular joints.

In a knee replacement, the surgeon makes thin cuts on the ends of the thighbone (femur) and shin bone (tibia) where the two bones meet and caps them with metal implants, placing a small plastic spacer in between. A thick piece of plastic mounted onto the tibial implant (in the shin) serves the function of cartilage, allowing for smooth, flowing movement. The back of the kneecap is fitted with a small plastic disc (see Figure 2, above right).

With hip replacement, the surgeon removes the

Figure 2: Total knee replacement

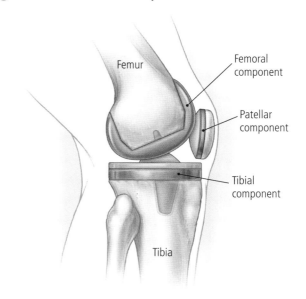

The surgeon first cuts away thin slices of bone with damaged cartilage from the bottom end of the femur and the top of the tibia, making sure that the bones are cut to precisely fit the shape of replacement pieces. The artificial joint is attached to the bones with cement or screws. A small plastic piece goes on the back of the kneecap (patella) to ride smoothly over the other parts of the artificial joint when you bend your knee.

head of the thighbone and replaces it with an artificial ball (the femoral component). The ball fits into a titanium cup that is placed in the hip (the acetabular cup; see Figure 3, page 12). There is a hard plastic (polyethylene) interface between them to allow smooth movement.

A new knee or hip won't necessarily give you more mobility, but it can take away the pain that holds you back. Replacing a diseased joint with an artificial one brings many people relief from pain and a renewed ability to engage in daily activities, after they have recovered from the procedure. However, there are also downsides to consider, including the pain of the surgery, the potential of a long recovery, and the chance of complications (see "Possible complications of joint replacement," page 13). Also, artificial joints can wear out in 10 to 20 years, depending on your weight and activity level, so you may eventually need a second surgery to replace them.

The decision about whether and when to replace

Figure 3: Hip replacement surgery

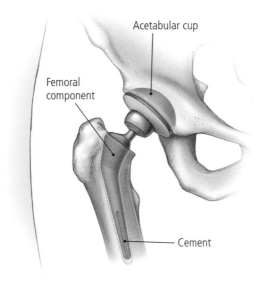

When rough and damaged cartilage prevents the bones of the hip from moving smoothly, an orthopedic surgeon can install an artificial joint with two parts. The head of the femur (thighbone) is replaced with an artificial ball with a long stem (the femoral component) that fits down inside the femur. An artificial cup, called the acetabular cup, fits inside the hip socket. The two pieces fit smoothly together to restore comfortable ball-in-socket movement.

a joint is not a simple one, and replacement is recommended only after more conservative options have been tried. You are a good candidate for joint replacement if you meet all of these criteria:

- You have pain that interferes with daily tasks and simple movements like walking and sitting, and the arthritis is taking a physical, mental, and emotional toll.
- X-rays of the joint show significant damage and cartilage loss.
- Other treatments have failed or cause unpleasant side effects.

Keep in mind that a joint replacement is an elective procedure, so there is no rush to decide. Take as much time as you need to talk with your doctor and surgeon about your options and to understand what's best for you. Some people prefer to manage joint pain conservatively for years with medications, wraps, and exercise, while others prefer to have surgery sooner, while they're still in good health, to reduce the risk of potential medical complications.

A variety of artificial joints are on the market, made from different materials and with different features. The joint replacement may be full or, in the knees, partial (using a smaller implant that leaves part of the original joint intact). The procedure may be performed with the traditional approach (using one large incision) or a minimally invasive one (using two or more smaller incisions).

Different incision locations can also be used. Most often, the surgeon will cut into the hip either from the back (posterior hip replacement) or from the front (anterior hip replacement). In the posterior approach, the surgeon has the best view of the joint, but needs to cut through the gluteus maximus muscle in the buttock, leading to a longer recovery time and a slightly higher dislocation rate. In the anterior approach, the surgeon works in between muscle layers, but has a more limited view, making the surgery more technically challenging. Many surgeons specialize in one approach or another, but you can make the decision together.

The surgery itself generally takes one or two hours. You may receive general anesthesia or, alternatively, a combination of a nerve block of the lower half of your body (to prevent pain and stop you from moving during the surgery) plus a sedating anesthetic like propofol (so you aren't aware of what's going on). The total hospital stay is usually around one to two days but varies depending on your health status and the type of procedure. Healthy, younger people may be candidates for same-day procedures, which cost less and reduce the risk of acquiring an infection in the hospital.

If you need to have both hips (or both knees) replaced, this can be done in two separate surgeries several months apart, but it is also possible to have both joints replaced at the same time. The benefits of simultaneous replacement are a single anesthesia, shorter total hospitalization, and one rehabilitation that allows you to resume normal activities sooner. However, having two joints replaced at the same time increases the risk of some complications; for example, there is a slightly elevated risk of blood clots and increased blood loss that may require transfusion.

Prehabilitation. One of the best things you can do for a successful joint replacement is to make your joint as strong and healthy as possible beforehand. Studies have found that "prehabilitation"—six weeks or so of cardio, strength, and functional exercises performed under the guidance of a physical therapist before a procedure like joint replacement surgery—can help prevent pain, speed your recovery, get you out of the hospital faster, and reduce the number of postsurgical rehab sessions you may need. Many clinical centers now offer water- and land-based "pre-hab" programs.

Presurgical education. Another key to a successful outcome in joint replacement surgery is knowing what to expect. Presurgical education programs explain the mechanics of the hip or knee and how the joint will be replaced, and they prepare you for what will happen on the day of surgery and immediately afterward, including pain management and rehabilitation. They also explain what you need to do to prepare yourself and your home, so you can manage in the days and weeks afterward. These programs are typically run by a physical therapist affiliated with your surgeon. They are usually offered in person at the hospital or outpatient center where you will have your surgery, but during the COVID-19 pandemic, they have been held online. Typically there is one session, and there is no separate charge for it. For more information about some of the topics that are covered, see "Preparing for surgery," page 14.

Recovering from joint replacement

In the past, people often rested for days or weeks in the hospital after joint replacement surgery, but new strategies have helped people regain mobility much faster.

"Enhanced recovery" or "fast-track" programs help people get back on their feet the same day as joint replacement surgery and leave the hospital that day or a day or two later. Programs usually accomplish this through a combination of patient education and preparation before the procedure, better use of pain medications after the operation (for example, a reduction in opioids, which cause nausea and grogginess), use of aspirin (instead of other blood thinners) for three weeks after the surgery in order to

Possible complications of joint replacement

The success rate for knee and hip replacement is very high. However, complications can occur that shorten the life of an implant, and you may need to take certain precautions.

Infection. Your implant can become infected soon after surgery or even years later. When it occurs later, it is almost always because infection elsewhere in the body has spread to the area. Seek immediate treatment if you have symptoms of an infection, particularly of the urinary tract, and inform all your doctors that you have a joint replacement.

Leg-length discrepancy. A difference in leg length occurs only rarely after knee replacement but occurs frequently, at least temporarily, after hip replacement. Before surgery, one leg is often shorter than the other—or feels shorter because the joint has deteriorated. Your orthopedic surgeon chooses an implant and plans surgery so that your legs will be equal in length after healing. After hip replacement, muscle weakness or spasm and swelling around the hip may temporarily cause an abnormal tilt to your pelvis and make you feel as though your legs are unequal in length. Stretching and strengthening exercises help restore your pelvis to its proper position. It may be several months before you can tell if the discrepancy is real and needs to be addressed with the use of a lift in one shoe.

Dislocation. In the weeks after a hip replacement, you'll need to take great care to keep from dislocating the implant before the surrounding tissues have healed enough to hold it in place. Even afterward, there is a chance of a painful dislocation—about four out of every 100 implants dislocate within 10 years of total hip replacement surgery, with the vast majority occurring within two months of the surgery. (The rate may be lower if your surgeon has cut into your body using an anterior rather than a posterior approach.) If your hip dislocates, you will need to go to the hospital emergency department, where you will be given a sedative and the implant ball will be manipulated back into the socket. A hip that dislocates more than once usually requires surgery to make the joint more stable.

Loosening. A replacement joint can loosen because the cement never secured it properly or eventually wore out, or because the surrounding bone remodeled over time, allowing the implant to loosen the tight attachment to bone. This may require a second surgery.

Bone loss. As a joint implant suffers wear and tear, loose particles can drift into the joint. As your immune system attacks these foreign particles, it can also attack surrounding bone, weakening it in a process called osteolysis. This, in turn, may loosen the bone's connection to the implant. Osteolysis is a major factor leading to the need for more surgery after hip and knee replacement, and it can occur with both cemented joints and uncemented joints.

prevent blood clots and also allow people to take ibuprofen or naproxen for pain relief (rather than relying on opioids), and encouragement in starting daily tasks and exercises as soon as possible. National studies have found a statistically significant decrease in complications following a total joint replacement with enhanced recovery programs.

For people on the fast track, rehabilitation begins the same day as surgery. For others, it will generally begin the next day. Often this will involve moving your leg around the joint with help from a physical therapist. The clinical staff will help you get out of bed and move around. Before you go home, you'll be asked to show that you can get in and out of bed without help; walk with a walker, cane, or crutches; and manage obstacles like steps that you may face at home. Directly after the procedure, you'll need assistance with daily tasks like shopping, cooking, and bathing.

Putting effort into your recovery is essential for long-term mobility with an artificial joint. See a physical therapist regularly after the procedure; over the next weeks and months, the more you engage in exercise—including light strength, balance, and gait training—the more successful your recovery will be. In

Preparing for surgery

Joint replacement can be highly successful, but to get the best results, you need to make preparations beforehand. These are the kinds of issues that are covered in presurgical education (see page 13).

Make arrangements

There are certain steps that are essential, including the following:

- Get clearance from your primary care doctor to have surgery. Primary care doctors typically don't know you're having orthopedic surgery unless you inform them of that fact. They will need to perform blood tests and often an electrocardiogram to make sure you are healthy enough to have surgery and tolerate anesthesia.

- Start performing preoperative exercises (see "Prehabilitation," page 12).

- Arrange for a family member or friend to stay with you for the immediate postoperative period and take care of any pets or children.

- Buy a cane or walker. (You'll receive crutches, if you need them, on the day of surgery from the physical therapist who works with you after the operation.)

- Apply for a temporary disabled parking permit through your state department of motor vehicles. Do this several weeks before your surgery.

Two other items are not easy to check off your list, but they can be a tremendous help to healing, if you are able to do them.

- Lose weight. Weight loss will help reduce pain and speed healing postoperatively. In fact, some surgeons refuse to perform elective surgeries like joint replacement on people who have a body mass index over 35, because of the increased risk of medical complications after surgery, including blood clots.

- Quit smoking. Many studies show that smokers have an increased risk of complications, including poor wound healing and pulmonary problems such as pneumonia.

Purchase assistive devices

You won't be able to move easily at first. The following purchases can help when you get home:

- Assistive devices—such as a grabber stick (to reach things without bending), a long-handled shoe horn, and a sock aid (to pull on your socks)—can help extend your reach.

- If you don't have one already, it's also a good idea to purchase an apron with big pockets to help you carry things around your home, while leaving your hands and arms free to use crutches or help you balance better.

Prepare your home

You will be grateful if you've already set up everything for maximum convenience and safety. The following will help:

- Arrange your bed so you have everything you need nearby, such as your cellphone, the TV remote control, tissues, medications, water, reading materials, and DVDs.

- Place other items you will need—clothing, toiletries, pots and pans, and so forth—at arm height.

- Do your grocery shopping prior to surgery.

- Prepare meals that you can freeze before the surgery and simply reheat as needed.

- Remove throw rugs, loose electrical cords, clutter, and other things you might trip over.

- Install night lights, so you can see at night if you have to get up to use the bathroom.

- Install grab bars in the bathroom (in the shower and by the toilet).

- Install a raised seat for the toilet.

addition to targeted exercises, you should gradually increase the distance you walk or the duration you are active so that you continue to challenge yourself. Just be careful to avoid activities like climbing stairs until you have enough strength and balance to manage them without injury (see "Dos and don'ts after joint replacement surgery," at right). By the first week or two, you should be walking with a cane. After a few weeks, you should no longer need the cane, and you may even be able to drive if you're not using opioids and your surgeon and physical therapist give you the all-clear. By three to six months, you should be functioning normally.

Osteoporosis and hip fractures

Mobility relies on bones that are strong enough to handle the physical demands of life, but osteoporosis can undermine this goal. It is a progressive and often insidious condition that can gradually weaken bones without causing noticeable symptoms—until you break a bone. Fractures are extremely common; half of all women and one-quarter of all men over age 50 will have an osteoporosis-related fracture at some point. The most common places to break a bone as a result of osteoporosis are the hip, spine, and wrist.

Particularly devastating are hip fractures, which account for about one in seven fractures resulting from osteoporosis. Many people who break a hip never fully regain their independence; about half need some kind of assistance walking, and one in four requires long-term care in a nursing home. The fracture itself is only part of the problem. Most people who expe-

▶ **Dos and don'ts after joint replacement surgery**

✘ **Don't soak your wound.** After returning from the hospital, keep your wound dry until it has thoroughly healed.

✔ **Do look for signs of infection.** These include persistent fever, shaking, chills, increasing redness or swelling of the knee or hip, drainage from the surgical site, and increasing pain with both activity and rest.

✔ **Do learn the signs of blood clots.** Joint replacement surgery carries a risk of potentially dangerous blood clots, and doctors routinely prescribe anti-clotting drugs like aspirin to prevent them from forming after surgery. Warning signs of a leg clot include increasing pain, tenderness, redness, or swelling in your knee and leg. Signs a clot has traveled to your lung include shortness of breath and chest pain that comes on suddenly with coughing. Call your doctor or seek immediate attention at an ER if you develop any of these signs.

✘ **Don't take risks that could cause you to fall.** Be especially careful on stairs. Use a cane, crutches, or a walker until your balance and strength have improved. You can climb stairs immediately, but only by leading with your good leg and going up one step at a time while holding on to the railing. Going down, lead with your operative leg. (Remember this mantra: Up with the good, down with the bad.)

✔ **Do be aware of movement restrictions after total hip replacement.** (There are no restrictions after total knee replacement.) For the first three months after surgery, it's important to observe the following rules to prevent your new hip from dislocating:

• Do keep the leg on the operated side facing forward.

• Don't cross your legs at the knees or bring your knee up higher than your hip.

• Don't bend at the waist beyond 90°.

• Don't lean forward while you're sitting or as you sit down.

• Don't pick things up from the floor while you're sitting (use a grabber stick).

• Don't turn your feet inward or outward when you bend down.

✔ **Do eat right.** Eating a healthy diet, including lots of fruits, vegetables, and whole grains, is important to promote proper tissue healing and restore muscle strength.

✔ **Do exercise wisely.** Performing the exercises your physical therapist recommends is crucial to restoring movement in your new joint and strengthening the surrounding muscles.

rience hip fractures are elderly, and many have other medical conditions that hamper their recovery. Medical complications from the fracture or the surgery to repair it can further erode health, putting people on a downward trajectory.

How does osteoporosis sneak up on you? Bones may seem inert, but like most other tissues in the body, they contain living cells and undergo continuous changes, in a process called remodeling. For example, when blood levels of calcium fall too low, cells called osteoclasts break down bone to release calcium for other uses through the body. Cells called osteoblasts then rebuild the bone's structure, so calcium and other minerals can accumulate again. Bones also become denser in response to weight-bearing exercise.

Early in life, bone accumulation exceeds bone loss because your body is growing. You reach peak bone density around age 27; it then levels off for about 10 years before beginning to decline, as bone demolition outpaces rebuilding. Eventually the bones become more porous, weaker, and more subject to fractures. Aging is the major risk factor for osteoporosis. In women, menopause leads to rapid bone loss.

In addition, with advancing age, the body tends to absorb less calcium from food and store it less efficiently elsewhere in the body, so it draws more on the body's "bank account" of calcium in the bones. To make matters worse, many people consume less calcium as they age. And aging bodies produce less vitamin D, which is important for helping the body absorb calcium from food and for creating new bone tissue. Moreover, many older people also exercise less, so bones do not receive the same signals from weight-bearing exercise to bulk up.

Finally, in addition to these normal changes, medical conditions such as cancer, liver disease, hyperparathyroidism (an overactive parathyroid gland), and anorexia can lead to osteoporosis. Some medications—including corticosteroids, proton-pump inhibitors, aromatase inhibitors for breast cancer, and androgen inhibitors for prostate cancer—can also promote bone loss or weakness. Your lifestyle and habits influence bone health, too: if you consume too little calcium and vitamin D, smoke cigarettes, drink too much alcohol, or don't get enough physical activity, you are at higher risk of developing osteoporosis. Among women, osteoporosis is more common in Caucasian and Asian women than in those of other ethnic backgrounds, and in women who are thin and small-boned or very low in body fat.

Preventing osteoporosis

While it's true that all people lose bone density as they age, it may never become full-blown osteoporosis, especially if you take steps to minimize bone loss.

Exercise. The best way to protect bone health is with regular exercise. When you put force on your bones, it prompts your body to strengthen those bones, so they can better withstand the stresses. Any type of exercise in which you lift weight or support your own weight can help. (Biking or swimming, while otherwise beneficial, do not.) Walking and hiking are good for keeping the bones in your legs and hips strong, although higher-impact activities like jogging or tennis have a more pronounced effect because the stresses on bone are greater.

Diet. Make sure your diet has all the nutrients it needs to keep building bone. In particular:

- **Calcium** is the main ingredient of bone. Dairy foods provide the most concentrated sources, but you can also find calcium in such foods as sockeye salmon, sardines, fortified orange juice, dried beans, nuts, and tofu made with calcium sulfate.
- **Vitamin D** helps the body absorb calcium. The body makes its own vitamin D when sunlight hits skin. Unfortunately, vitamin D is naturally found in only a few foods, such as salmon, tuna, mackerel, and fish liver oils. However, it's added to most milk in the United States and some other products, like breakfast cereals, orange juice, and yogurt.
- **Vitamin K** helps produce a protein involved in making bone. Studies have found that people who take in higher levels of vitamin K are less likely to break their hips. Vitamin K is found in broccoli, brussels sprouts, leafy greens, and cabbage.

Whether you get these nutrients from foods or from supplements will depend somewhat on your diet and your health risks (see "Do you need supplements?" on page 46).

Bone-building medications. Medications can also play a key role, including

- bisphosphonates, such as alendronate (Fosamax), ibandronate (Boniva), risedronate (Actonel), and zoledronic acid (Reclast)
- estrogen (Premarin, Estrace, others)
- the selective estrogen receptor modulator raloxifene (Evista)
- the monoclonal antibody denosumab (Prolia). ▼

A good foundation: Feet and ankles

Your feet are literally the foundation of your mobility. They have a complex structure with over 50 bones combined and even more joints, all designed to manage pressure, weight, and force, while being extremely flexible. Each foot consists of three basic parts: the forefoot (the toes and ball of your foot), the midfoot (the arch), and the hindfoot (the heel).

Foot pain can arise at any age, but many of the problems that emerge in feet are the result of wear and tear or lifelong habits like wearing uncomfortable shoes, so they become more frequent with age. Chronic foot pain is a common complaint of seniors and one of the reasons many people limit their movement with age. Foot problems can also lead to falls, and thus to broken bones, which can be disastrous for mobility.

Figure 4: Sites where structural problems occur

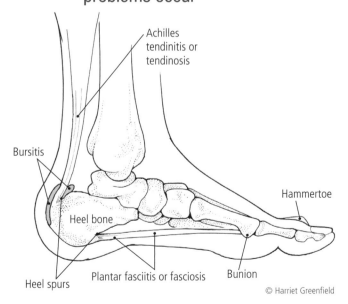

© Harriet Greenfield

The foot is a complex structure and can experience a variety of structural problems or injuries. Among the more common of these are Achilles tendinitis, Achilles tendinosis, bursitis, plantar fasciitis or fasciosis, heel spurs, bunions and bunionettes, and hammertoes.

Common foot problems

Feet are subject to a host of problems (see Figure 4, below left), but following are the ones that most frequently limit mobility.

Achilles tendinitis and Achilles tendinosis. Heel pain may occur when the Achilles tendon, which runs up the back of the heel, suffers damage, inflammation, or degeneration. With Achilles tendinitis, the tendon becomes inflamed. A separate but related problem, Achilles tendinosis, occurs when the tendon degrades—much like a rope fraying. Because the symptoms and treatment of these two problems are virtually the same, you may not know whether you have Achilles tendinitis or tendinosis, or both, unless you ask your doctor. But it's good to know, because if you develop Achilles tendinosis, it's vital that you take steps to protect your tendon from further structural damage. The tendon can be damaged by overexertion from running or other high-impact activities, weight gain, or wearing ill-fitting shoes.

These conditions are usually treated with a combination of approaches, including the RICE first-aid regimen (see "RICE for injuries," page 6), pain relievers, and light stretching exercises. Special night splints and footwear inserts can also provide relief.

Bunions and bunionettes. A bunion often looks like a growth on the side of the foot at the base of the big toe. But it is actually a misalignment of the bones that causes the big toe to turn inward, toward (or sometimes under) the other toes. Bunions are among the most common toe problems and are more common in women than in men. A bunionette is a similar condition that affects the base of the smallest toe.

Because the most frequent cause of bunions and bunionettes is wearing shoes with cramped toe boxes, wearing roomier shoes is the best step to take to prevent them from forming (see "Shoes: What to wear?" on page 18). Roomy shoes, shoe inserts, and special pads can also help relieve pain, as can hot and cold

Shoes: What to wear?

The shoes you choose to wear every day have a cumulative effect on the health of your feet. Crowded, ill-fitting shoes can lead to blisters, bunions, corns, calluses, hammertoes, and other painful problems. High heels can cause foot problems as well as back pain, postural misalignment, shortened calf muscles, and falls. Fortunately, there are many shoes available today designed for both comfort and style.

Look for shoes with a wide toe box that doesn't squeeze your toes together. Women are especially prone to buying shoes that are too small, and the vast majority of foot problems in women come from wearing tight shoes. One helpful tip is to shop for shoes in the afternoon when your feet have expanded slightly, to keep you from choosing too-tight shoes. Wear the socks or stockings that you would expect to wear with the shoes. Don't be shy about asking to get your foot measured by a salesperson—most people's feet get slightly larger and wider as they age, so your size may need adjustment over time.

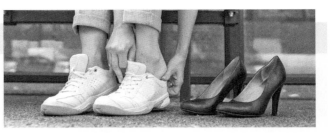

© AndreyPopov | Getty Images

Also make sure the shoe offers plenty of cushioning and support, including built-in arch supports. Many shoes today are designed with memory foam and composite soles to offer extra shock absorption. When looking for athletic shoes, always choose shoes that are designed for the activity you'll be doing. Make sure they are roomy enough so that your toes don't hit the front of the shoe as you move.

For daily use, women should opt for shoes with a low heel—no higher than three-quarters of an inch. The higher the heel, the worse it will be for your feet, even if the heels are wide.

For the names of shoe manufacturers that have earned the American Podiatric Medical Association's Seal of Acceptance, visit www.apma.org.

---

compresses. In severe cases, surgery called proximal metatarsal osteotomy realigns the bones (see Figure 5, page 19), but it is a major procedure that requires at least three months for recovery.

Hammertoes. Another cause of toe pain is a hammertoe, a deformity that develops when tendons and ligaments in a toe contract, causing the toe to bend over and curl up—resembling a hammer. The top of your toe may then rub against your shoe, causing irritation, corns, calluses, or even bursitis. The problem usually develops in the second toe, often because a bunion has formed in the big toe, forcing it inward and displacing the second toe. Shoes with narrow toe boxes, which compress the toes, increase the risk for a hammertoe. Usually hammertoes are flexible at first; that is, if you apply pressure to the toe, it will flatten back down. But over time, a hammertoe can become rigid and may become more painful and inflamed.

You can relieve hammertoe pain by applying ice or cold compresses or by soaking your foot in warm water. For severe cases, surgery may be necessary.

Bursitis. A bursa is a fluid-filled sac that cushions a tendon near a bone. If a bursa becomes inflamed, the painful condition is known as bursitis.

To prevent bursitis at the back of the heel, make sure that your shoes fit correctly and provide plenty of cushioning. The condition is generally treated like Achilles tendinitis, with the RICE regimen (see "RICE for injuries," page 6) and nonprescription pain relievers. Bursitis can take from six to 12 months to heal.

Osteoarthritis of the feet. If osteoarthritis develops in your toes or other foot bones, it can cause pain and stiffness in your feet and can affect your normal gait, causing you to favor one side or limp. Obesity and previous foot injuries are major risk factors for foot osteoarthritis.

The condition can be alleviated with gentle stretching exercises like the ones in this chapter (see "Exercises and stretches for your feet and ankles," page 21). You can reduce pain and any inflammation with hot and cold packs, NSAIDs, or the COX-2 inhibitor celecoxib (Celebrex). Your doctor may also recommend shoe inserts to adjust your walking gait in a way that will take pressure off aching joints. If these strategies don't alleviate your arthritis pain, surgery to repair or replace damaged joints may be necessary. To help protect your feet from injury—which in turn can lead to osteoarthritis—wear well-fitting, well-built shoes with cushioned soles.

Calluses and corns. Calluses are broad areas of

thick skin that usually form on the bottom of the feet as a protective response against the wear and tear of walking, a structural abnormality in the feet, or shoes that rub. Corns are smaller, hard growths and usually develop on the tops or sides of toes; softer ones may also develop between toes. They often arise from wearing tight shoes. Some hardening of the skin on feet is normal, but sometimes it leads to pain or trouble walking.

Better-fitting shoes will reduce the irritation that caused the problem in the first place, and over time, the corns or calluses will shrink on their own. But don't expect overnight results; the process will take weeks or even months. If you can't wait that long, you can treat the problem on your own, unless you have diabetes, peripheral neuropathy, or a circulatory problem; in those cases, you should never try to treat a corn or callus yourself, or you may develop an infection. Assuming you don't have any of these conditions, you can remove dead skin by soaking feet in warm water and gently rubbing the area with a pumice stone or foot file. Afterward, moisturize the area with skin lotion. For larger corns and calluses, consult a foot care specialist, who will shave away some of the thickened skin.

Plantar fasciitis. The plantar fascia is a strong band of tissue on the underside of the foot that connects the ball of your foot to the heel. It's highly susceptible to becoming irritated and inflamed, and this condition— plantar fasciitis—is a common cause of heel pain.

Plantar fasciitis may get better on its own, but you may be able to speed healing. When pain comes on, lightly stretch the foot and ice it. Taking NSAIDs can help control pain and inflammation. Physical therapy for plantar fasciitis, which includes a program of exercises to stretch the heel and bottom of the foot, can also help. Physical therapists also sometimes pair exercises with extracorporeal shock wave therapy, which uses high-energy sound waves to reduce pain, or laser therapy. The exact way these procedures work is unknown and they haven't been studied extensively, but they may still be helpful.

Gout. Gout is a form of arthritis that occurs when uric acid, a normal byproduct of digestion, accumulates in the joints and forms crystals. The big toe is a common site for symptoms, which include stabbing pain, redness, and swelling. Gout is more common in men than women, but in women the risk goes up after age 50, because uric acid levels increase after menopause. Certain foods with high levels of substances called purines (including anchovies, sardines, mussels, scallops, lentils, and red and organ meats) can raise uric acid levels.

Gout is usually treated with pain relievers, steroid injections, prescription medications, and changes in the diet.

Diabetic foot damage. Diabetes can damage both the blood vessels and the nerves that serve the feet. Because nerve damage impairs pain sensation, a foot injury can go unnoticed, worsen, and become a feeding ground for invasive bacteria. Poor circulation makes the problem worse by impeding the body's infection-fighting cells. If not treated, foot ulcers can penetrate deep below the skin and spread infection into bone.

The best way of treating diabetic foot injuries is by avoiding them in the first place. To minimize the chances of injuring your feet, avoid going barefoot. Wear well-fitting, comfortable shoes that offer good

Figure 5: Surgical correction of a bunion

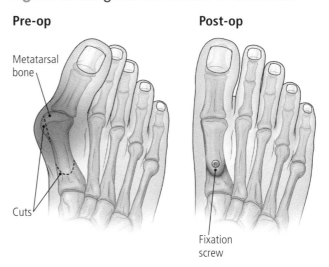

To correct a bunion, a surgeon can use one of several procedures in which the enlarged portion of the bone is shaved off.

The procedure illustrated here, known as a proximal metatarsal osteotomy, is used to correct a severe bunion. First, the surgeon cuts away a portion of the bunion at the head of the metatarsal bone. Next, he or she cuts the lower portion of the same bone and rotates it to correct the bone alignment. A pin or screw fastens the bone segments.

protection, and wear clean socks every day. You should also examine your feet every day for cuts, sores, or scratches, so that you can treat any wounds immediately. Have all calluses, corns, warts, and other foot ailments treated by a podiatrist.

Keeping feet healthy

Feet are easy to neglect. But taking a few simple steps to care for your feet should be part of your overall strategy for maintaining mobility.

Maintain a healthy weight. Being overweight affects your feet by putting greater force on them with each step. It can increase your risk of having a condition like arthritis in the feet, and it can worsen pain from other foot problems. Being overweight can also harm foot health by putting you at higher risk for diabetes or poor blood circulation, which can lead to foot pain and loss of sensation in the feet.

Wear good shoes. Many of the common foot problems that are described in this chapter result from wearing tight, poorly fitting shoes, especially high heels. One survey conducted by the American Podiatric Medical Association found that 49% of women wear high heels—and three-quarters of them report that the shoes cause them pain. A lifetime of wearing comfortable shoes is one of the best preventive measures you can take to ensure your mobility.

Moisturize your feet. The skin of the feet tends to get thinner and drier with age; calloused feet can crack and bleed, causing pain. To keep the skin soft, rub a thick moisturizing lotion into your feet after showers or baths as needed. Avoid the spaces in between the toes, where moisture can lead to bacterial overgrowth.

> ### ▶ Helpful hint
>
> As people grow older, their toenails often become thicker, making them harder to cut. Here's a home remedy that works: apply a bit of Vicks VapoRub ointment (normally used for easing chest congestion) to your thick nails, massaging it on gently. Wipe off any excess ointment before pulling on socks or going to bed. After a month or so of daily applications, you should find your toenails softer and easier to trim.

Practice good foot hygiene. Wash and dry your feet thoroughly when you shower or bathe. Cut toenails straight across to avoid ingrown nails (see "Helpful hint," below left). Use a pumice stone or foot file to gently remove calluses. If you wear nail polish, let the toenails "breathe" for a couple of days after you remove it and before adding more, to keep nails healthy.

Stretch your feet. People don't usually think about stretching the tops and bottoms of their feet, but stretches can help you treat—and prevent—foot pain. Stretches for the Achilles tendon are also important (see "Exercises and stretches for your feet and ankles," page 21).

Active ankles

Your ankles make important contributions to movement. The ankle is a joint made of three bones: the tibia (shin bone), the fibula (a thin bone that runs parallel to the tibia on the outside of the leg), and the talus (the central ankle bone that sits at the top of the foot). The bony bumps you feel on the inside and outside of the ankle are part of the tibia and fibula. The talus sits between these two bumps and works like a hinge to allow you to point and flex your foot. The ankle also has joints to permit sideways movement.

Ankle sprains, which involve the stretching or tearing of ligaments in the ankle joint, are extremely common. Whenever you land improperly on your feet and your ankle rolls to one side or twists, it can cause a sprain. The setback is usually temporary, but frequent sprains can cause long-term problems.

Ankle sprains are more common in people who have loose ligaments or weak ankle muscles. Both make the ankle more likely to twist or bend accidentally. A poor sense of balance—including any problems in sensing touch or the position of your foot in space—can contribute to sprains and falls. Sprains should be treated with the RICE method (see "RICE for injuries," page 6). Exercises to strengthen your ankles and preserve balance can help you prevent sprains (see "Balance exercises," page 34).

Some people develop osteoarthritis of the ankle, particularly ballet dancers who have subjected their ankles to years of stress, or people with foot condi-

Exercises and stretches for your feet and ankles

Exercising and stretching your feet and ankles is often a component of physical therapy for foot pain; it's also a good practice to maintain mobility in your feet and ankles. These simple stretching exercises can be done as a short addition to your daily routine.

Limber up

1. Sit in a chair with your feet flat on the floor.

2. Lift your left leg so your foot is off the floor and use your big toe to make circles in the air, moving in a clockwise direction, for 15 to 20 rotations.

3. Reverse direction and make another 15 to 20 circles, this time in a counterclockwise direction.

4. Repeat with your right foot.

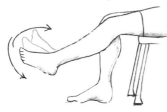

Bottom-of-foot stretch

1. Stand with your feet together.

2. Step back with your left leg so your heel is raised and your toes press against the ground. You should feel the muscles on the bottom of your feet pull gently.

3. Hold for 20 to 30 seconds.

4. Repeat with your right foot.

Top-of-foot stretch

1. Stand with your feet together.

2. Now, working with one foot at a time, raise your left heel and curl your toes under, pressing the tops of your toes against the floor. You should feel the muscles on the top of your foot and the front of your ankle gently stretch.

3. Hold for 20 to 30 seconds.

4. Repeat with the right foot.

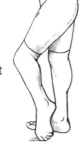

Achilles tendon (runner's) stretch

1. Stand at arm's length from a wall, pressing your hands against it and keeping your feet together.

2. Step back with your left leg, bending your right knee slightly and keeping the left heel on the ground. You should feel a stretch along your calf to your ankle.

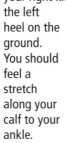

3. Hold for 20 to 30 seconds.

4. Repeat with your right leg.

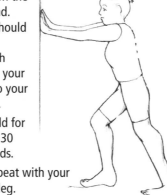

Ankle strength

1. Sit in a chair with your feet flat on the floor, pointing forward.

2. Lift your left leg. Hold the ends of an exercise band and place the center of the band under the ball of your left foot.

3. Slowly press against the exercise band, as if you were stepping on a pedal, and hold for a few seconds. You should feel a stretch on the upper part of your foot. Then release.

4. Repeat 10 to 15 times.

5. Repeat with your right leg.

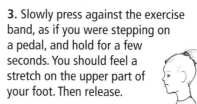
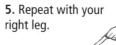

Heel exercises

1. Loop an exercise band around the leg of a heavy piece of furniture, such as a table or desk.

2. Sitting directly in front of it, slip your left foot into the loop so the exercise band curls around your forefoot, just below your toes.

3. Pull back with your forefoot, flexing at the ankle. Hold for several seconds, then relax. You should feel a stretch along the back of your heel.

4. Repeat 10 to 15 times.

5. Repeat with your right foot.

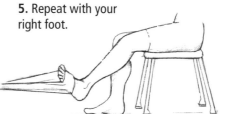

tions that put an extra burden on ankles. Special ankle braces, boots, or shoe inserts can ease the pain of ankle arthritis. Ankles are not surgically replaced as often as hips and knees, but new joint implants have improved over the past few years and the surgery is becoming more common. Severe cases of ankle arthritis may also be treated with surgery that fuses two bones together.

Exercises to improve ankle strength and flexibility are an important addition to the exercises for hips and knees, to maintain your mobility or to improve ankle strength. Exercising your ankles also builds your sensory awareness of these essential joints, making you less likely to fall or twist an ankle (see "Exercises and stretches for your feet and ankles," above). ♥

A stable support: Your back and posture

Your hips, legs, and feet make walking possible, but a healthy spine and the ability to maintain good posture are also essential to maintaining mobility and independence. The spine and the muscles that support it hold your body upright and give you the stability to do all your daily activities, even something as simple as standing and walking across the room.

Figure 6: Regions of the spine

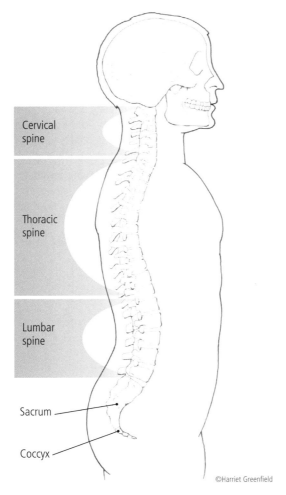

Cervical spine

Thoracic spine

Lumbar spine

Sacrum

Coccyx

©Harriet Greenfield

Your spine is divided into three regions: the cervical, the thoracic, and the lumbar. Low back pain originates in the lumbar area, which extends from the bottom of your rib cage to your sacrum (the triangular bone found between your hip bones).

Although we often think of a "straight back" as good posture, the spine can be divided into three areas, each of which has a gentle curve (see Figure 6, below left). These curves make it easier for the back to support the weight of the body, but if they become too exaggerated, movement becomes much more difficult.

Your spine may seem simple, but it has a remarkable design. Vertebrae, discs, ligaments, muscles, and nerves form a complex structure that enables you to twist, turn, bend, stand, walk, and lift. But the back's complexity also makes it vulnerable. In particular, the lower part of the spine supports much of your body's weight and is subjected to great stresses.

Back pain can be a sign of problems in the soft tissue, such as a muscle strain or a spinal disc that bulges out from its normal position or ruptures (herniates), putting pressure on nerves that branch out of the spinal cord. Or the pain could be a sign of compression fractures in the vertebrae resulting from osteoporosis (see "Compression fractures," page 25). The spine is particularly vulnerable to developing osteoporosis, because the main component of vertebrae is a spongy type of bone that is easily weakened. Spinal stenosis (see page 25)—a narrowing of the spinal canal—is another common cause of back pain in people over age 50. And, like other joints in the body, the spinal joints can develop osteoarthritis.

Back pain is a top reason that people begin to lose mobility in middle age. If it becomes chronic, it can keep you from being active and remaining fully engaged in your life. When something goes wrong in the spine, it can also cause numbness, weakness, or loss of movement in the areas the nerves supply.

Sprains and strains

The most common cause for sudden, temporary back pain is a sprain or strain due to overuse, unaccustomed activity, excessive lifting, or an accident of some kind.

Sprains affect ligaments, the tough, fibrous bands of tissue found where bones, such as the vertebrae in your spine, connect at joints. Strains are injuries of your muscles or your tendons, which connect muscles to bones.

Sprains and strains are usually relieved by over-the-counter pain medications and generally clear up in days or weeks. An ice pack applied immediately following the injury can also help by numbing the area and preventing or reducing swelling caused by inflammation. Use it on and off for 20 minutes at a time, but never apply ice directly to skin. Always wrap it in a towel to prevent frostbite. After 48 hours, applying heat may be more helpful, to warm and soothe aching muscles and increase blood flow (see "Heat for long-term pain and stiffness," page 7). Limit bed rest during the day to a few hours; lack of movement can actually postpone recovery.

If you're experiencing back pain that is intense or lasts more than a couple of weeks, see your doctor to get a proper diagnosis; x-rays and other imaging tests can help determine if there's underlying damage to the vertebrae or discs.

Exercise, posture, and other back-healthy habits

Pain from sprains and strains can keep you from engaging in physical activity, making it more difficult to maintain a healthy weight and keep up your strength, stamina, and balance as you age. So treating and managing back pain is crucial for staying on the path of a healthy and active life.

Whether you're experiencing a single episode of back pain or a chronic problem, you should try to stay active unless your doctor says not to. Even in the case of temporary muscle strains, bed rest can make the problem worse as the muscles that support your spine become weak and stiff from lack of use.

In fact, rehabilitative exercise can help lessen chronic low back pain for many people. Weak back and abdominal muscles, resulting from deconditioning or age, cause or worsen many cases of low back pain. Stretching and strengthening these muscles is important not only for treating low back pain, but also for preventing the problem from returning. (See "Strengthening your core," page 29, for one simple strengthening exercise.)

There is evidence that practicing yoga can help too. But yoga classes and instructors are highly variable, and yoga can also injure your back if you overstretch or push yourself into difficult poses—so opt for a class that is gentle, and modify poses as needed to avoid injury.

Any exercise program for back pain should be customized to meet your needs and introduced gradually. One universal rule about any exercise plan is to stop if it becomes painful. Exercise is meant to help, not hurt. If you were exercising before an episode of back pain and then had to slow down or stop for a while because of the pain, don't resume exercising at the same level as before the episode. Deconditioning occurs quickly; if you try to pick up your exercise routine where you left off, you might get hurt. Start by doing less (fewer minutes or fewer repetitions) and gradually build back up to where you were before.

Good posture when exercising, as well as in your daily life, not only prevents injuries but also helps you condition the muscles that keep you upright and supported in your everyday activity. It's helpful to use a mirror at first to check your posture and alignment. Good posture when standing means

- your chin parallel to the floor
- shoulders rolled back and down evenly
- arms at your sides, elbows relaxed and even
- abdominal muscles pulled in
- weight evenly placed over your hips and feet (not leaning to one side or another)
- your knees and feet pointing straight ahead.

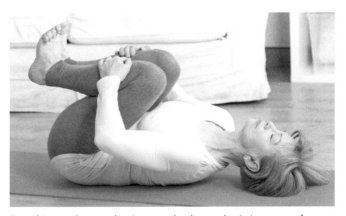

Stretching and strengthening your back muscles is important for treating low back pain. But any exercise program for back pain should be customized to meet your needs and introduced gradually.

Good posture can help not only when you're exercising, but also when you're carrying out everyday tasks, such as lifting things (see Figure 7, below).

In addition, you can take some of the pressure off your back by following some simple steps:

- While standing to perform ordinary tasks like chopping vegetables or folding laundry, keep one foot on a small step stool.
- When sitting, keep your knees a bit higher than your hips and bend them at a 90° angle. Sit with your feet comfortably on the floor. If your feet don't reach the floor, put a book or small stool under them.
- Don't remain seated or standing in the same position for too long. Stretch, shift your position, or take a short walk. Make frequent stops when driving long distances.
- Sleep on your side if you can, and bend your knees toward your chest a bit. Choose a pillow that keeps your head and neck in the same alignment they have when you're standing; overly thick or thin pillows that prop your head up too high or let it droop can distort your spine.
- Choose a mattress that's firm enough to support your spine but also follows your body's contours. Very soft mattresses pose the risk that you might sink in so deeply that your joints twist and become painful during the night. For older people, a soft mattress may also make it harder to get up and out of bed easily for late-night trips to the bathroom.

Nerve-compression syndromes

After sprains and strains, the next most common category of low back pain consists of conditions involving compressed nerves (often referred to as "pinched" nerves). Two major examples are disc problems (such as a herniated disc) and spinal stenosis, which occurs when a narrowing of the spinal column puts pressure on nerves in the spine.

Disc abnormalities

As a disc degenerates over time, its gelatinous center tends to dry out. The layers of the disc's outer shell often become thin and weak and start to tear, especially in the parts of the disc closest to the nerve roots. The disc can bulge like an underinflated tire and can herniate (meaning that the inner core of the disc protrudes from the outer shell). People commonly refer to this as a "slipped disc" or "ruptured disc."

This kind of pressure usually causes inflamma-

Figure 7: The laws of lifting

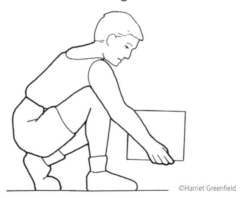

©Harriet Greenfield

Follow these steps when you lift something heavy:

1. Face the object and position yourself close to it.
2. Bend at your knees, not your waist, and squat down as far as you comfortably can.
3. Tighten your stomach and keep your buttocks tucked in.
4. Lift with your legs, not your back muscles.
5. Don't try to lift the object too high. Don't raise a heavy load any higher than your waist; keep even a light load below shoulder level.
6. Keep the object close to you as you lift it.
7. If you need to turn to set something down, don't twist your upper body. Instead, turn your entire body, moving your shoulders, hips, and feet at the same time.
8. Ask for help with lifting anything that's too heavy.

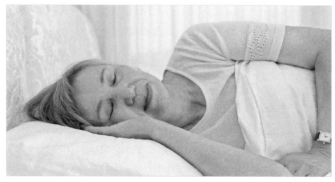

© baona | Getty Images

Try to keep your neck in a neutral position most of the time, including while you sleep. Choose a pillow that keeps your head and neck in the same alignment as when you're standing.

tion and back pain, often accompanied by sciatica—a sharp pain that runs along the path of the sciatic nerve, which passes through the buttock, down the leg, and into the foot.

Disc problems take longer to heal than simple sprains and strains. But 90% of people with sciatica or herniated discs will recover on their own within six months. For chronic pain, the best approach is a program combining pain-relieving medication, physical activity, and a complementary therapy such as acupuncture. If the pain still persists, your doctor may refer you to a pain clinic. These centers use a variety of approaches, including cognitive behavioral therapy, exercise programs, biofeedback, relaxation techniques, and selective nerve blocks to ease the pain or minimize its effect on your daily routine.

Spinal stenosis

The spinal cord runs through spaces in the vertebrae. If these spaces narrow for any reason—a condition called spinal stenosis—this puts pressure on the spinal cord and the spinal nerve roots. When it occurs in the lower spine, it can cause pain in the back or legs and can impair your mobility.

Nearly half of people in their 60s have some spinal stenosis in the lower back. It's the leading reason people get spinal surgery at that age. Symptoms include pain that begins in the buttocks and radiates down the legs (sciatica) and sometimes back pain. You might notice numbness and tingling in those areas, or even just weakness and fatigue. You may feel pain or cramping when standing for a long time or walking, and the pain usually lessens when you're seated—particularly if you lean forward, which allows the spine to stretch out. (In contrast, many other types of lower back pain feel worse with long periods of sitting.) Activities that involve leaning on a support—such as pushing a grocery cart or riding a bicycle—also feel less painful.

The condition can be treated with surgery, but most physicians recommend trying conservative treatments first. Medications such as NSAIDs can reduce inflammation and pain. Muscle relaxants, opioid medications, the antiseizure drug gabapentin (Neurontin), and some antidepressants, like amitriptyline (Elavil), are sometimes prescribed. Use these drugs only under a doctor's supervision, as they can have potentially harmful side effects, such as dampening breathing during sleep. As with other types of joint pain, occasional injections of corticosteroids may help by quelling inflammation.

Physical therapy can't heal the narrowing of the spinal column, but it can improve the spine's overall strength and flexibility, and it may help with managing pain and numbness from the condition. If you're struggling with spinal stenosis, adopting a regular exercise schedule that includes walking and light stretching can help you preserve your mobility as you work with your doctor to treat the condition.

When conservative treatments don't work, a procedure called decompression laminectomy is an option. It involves removing a thin piece of bone called the lamina at the back part of an affected vertebra to reduce pressure on the spinal cord. Spinal fusion, which entails use of a bone graft taken from the hip or pelvis to fuse two vertebrae together, is another option. It is usually performed together with decompression laminectomy in advanced cases to prevent spinal instability. It is controversial in some cases, however.

A third option, called interspinous spacer implantation, uses small metal devices implanted between spinous processes—the projections of the vertebrae that form the bumps close to your skin along your spine—in order to reduce the pressure on spinal nerves. Although the procedure is minimally invasive with a quick recovery time, people who have spacer implants are more likely to need surgery again.

Compression fractures

Unlike other fractures, compression fractures of the spine are not necessarily the result of a fall or another type of accident, although they can be. Rather, they occur more often when too much weight bears down on vertebrae that have been weakened by osteoporosis. Rather than snapping, the front of a vertebra collapses. Viewed from the side, vertebrae with compression fractures often look like wedges rather than level discs. Compression fractures can cause a person to lose height as the spine shrinks or to develop a hunched posture (see "Hyperkyphosis," page 26).

Some spinal fractures cause little or no pain, and the

only symptoms are the effects on the shape of the spine. In other cases, they can cause pain that is either sharp or dull and may radiate around the side of the body. They can also provoke spasms in muscles around the spine.

Spinal fractures can take a major toll on mobility. Over time, posture becomes distorted, and the core muscles that normally keep the body upright become weak. People with spinal fractures can have difficulty walking and maintaining balance and may rely on a cane or walker to move around (see "Mobility aids," page 7).

The standard treatment has long been to wait it out while the fractured bone heals. This process takes six weeks on average and is very painful; often people need narcotic painkillers or equivalent medications, such as tramadol (Ultram), a narcotic-like painkiller thought to be less addictive than narcotics.

In people with osteoporosis, either of two procedures—vertebroplasty or kyphoplasty—is sometimes used to treat compression fractures of the vertebrae. Both involve injecting surgical cement into the compressed vertebra to fill holes and crevices. But there are no large trials yet that confirm that these techniques are effective.

Hyperkyphosis

You may have seen someone, or even know someone, whose back hunches over in an exaggerated way. This condition is often referred to as a "dowager's hump," but in medical terminology, it's known as age-related postural hyperkyphosis. The problem is more than cosmetic: it can limit mobility and raise the risk of falls and fractures.

People with this condition are more likely to have trouble getting out of a chair without using their hands, have poorer balance, walk more slowly up stairs, and have a slowed or abnormal gait. They report greater difficulties with daily tasks like housework and an overall lower quality of life. Over time, the abnormal posture can lead to further joint problems, a higher risk of fractures, and difficulty breathing properly, since the bent posture leaves less room in the chest cavity for the lungs to inflate.

It isn't completely clear why some people begin to

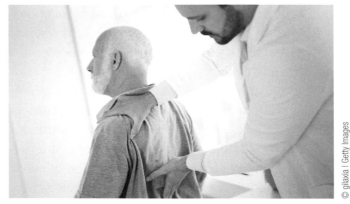

© gilaxia | Getty Images

Weakness in the muscles and connective tissues that hold the body upright can lead to a stooped posture. Targeted exercises designed to strengthen postural muscles and improve flexibility can help.

hunch over. In some cases, weakening or degeneration of the bones is to blame. Many people who have the condition have also experienced compression fractures (page 25). In other cases, weakness in the muscles and connective tissues that hold the body upright can also cause hyperkyphosis. Age-related declines in sensory awareness—such as the sense of balance and the body's position in space—may also lead people to gradually fail to maintain proper posture.

There's no easy treatment for hyperkyphosis. Targeted exercises designed to strengthen postural muscles and improve flexibility can help. For example, back-extension exercises, which involve gentle backward bending of the spine, may provide a limited amount of help counteracting hyperkyphosis. By contrast, exercises that flex the spine—those with movements in which you bend forward or curl up, including abdominal curls—can put undue stress on the vertebrae and have been linked with higher rates of fractures in women with hyperkyphosis. Other treatments include wearing braces, wearing a special weighted vest, or applying therapeutic tape across the shoulder blades and upper back to encourage a more upright posture.

The best prevention for hyperkyphosis is to maintain good posture and strengthen the muscles in the abdomen and back. Some studies suggest that forms of exercise that promote flexibility in the back, such as tai chi and yoga, can help prevent the condition from developing. Since the health of your bones also contributes to the shape of your spine, protecting bone health and treating osteoporosis are also important. ▼

Masterful muscles

More than 600 muscles work together to allow you to accomplish all the movements you make every day. Yet a process called sarcopenia—a gradual decrease in muscle tissue—can rob you of muscle mass and strength. Older people who have lost muscle become increasingly frail, and previously effortless activities like lifting a trash bag, climbing stairs, vacuuming the house, or getting dressed can start to feel burdensome. Such individuals are more likely to injure themselves and less likely to recover easily. They depend more and more on others to do tasks they once accomplished themselves.

Between the ages of 30 and 70, the average person loses about 25% of his or her muscle mass. By age 90, another 25% has disappeared. The nerves that signal muscles to contract also can deteriorate with age. At the same time, fat tends to accumulate around muscle fibers, which can lead to mobility problems.

Sarcopenia poses a major threat to the independence of older adults. But while some muscle loss seems to be an inevitable part of aging (because it gets harder to build muscle as you get older), much can be done to halt or slow the decline. Resistance training can boost muscle strength and also reduce the amount of fat that accumulates around muscles. Even elderly people can prevent a great deal of muscle loss with a strength training program.

In fact, declining muscle strength may stem from lack of use as much as from the inevitable changes that accompany age. Maintaining your muscles is one of the most important steps you can take to ensure your mobility and independence in later life.

Building a strength training routine

Building your muscles through strength training can improve mobility at all ages and fitness levels. If you're already physically fit, increasing your strength training can help you maintain your muscle mass and performance as you age. If you have lost some of your mobil-ity, strength training may help you regain it—allowing you to use a cane instead of a walker, for instance, or maintain your walking speed for a longer period of time. It can help you accomplish tasks like lifting grocery bags or getting in and out of a car.

Generally speaking, anyone who is healthy or has a well-controlled heath problem, such as high blood pressure or diabetes, can safely do strength and power training. That includes frail older people. But some people will need more supervision or must observe more restrictions than others. Check with your doctor before embarking on a strength training program if you have a heart condition, a previous injury, a recent surgery, new pain or swelling, or any chronic diseases that could potentially be worsened by exercise.

There are endless ways to exercise effectively, so pick the approach that works best for you, based on your fitness level. The exercises described in this chapter (see "Three simple strength and power exercises," page 28) can be performed on your own with no special equipment. Other people prefer the structure of a gym, group exercise classes, or working with a personal trainer for motivation. But if you work with a personal trainer, be cautious. First, ask about his or her certification—the American College of Sports Medicine offers the most rigorous certification program. But this certification involves relatively little medical training, so even a well-meaning trainer can push you beyond your limits and put you at risk of injury. Make sure your trainer respects your body's capabilities.

To get the full benefits of strength training, you have to do it regularly—and keep it up over time—because the benefits start to disappear when you stop exercising. For this reason, it's important to choose a routine that you'll be able to stick with for the long haul. Aim for comfort, safety, and consistency, and rather than lifting as much weight as you possibly can, go for more repetitions with less weight to build stamina. The goal is to maintain your muscles, not to build a new physique. And you can forget the old adage "no pain, no gain." Aiming for too much weight too fast is more apt to lead to injury than health benefits. Avoid doing deep squats, lunges, and deep lifts with kettlebells; these are favorite exercises of many trainers, but they put pressure on your joints and can lead to injuries if you don't do them perfectly every time. Dr. Scott Martin, the medical editor of this report, says that among his patients, these three exercises are responsible for more back, hip, and knee injuries than any others.

It's a good idea to inform your doctor about any new training program to make sure it's appropriate. If you have a health condition or are recovering from an injury, consider seeing a physiatrist or physical therapist who can set you up with exercises that are safe and beneficial for your condition.

Aging and power training

Just as muscle mass and strength decline with age, so does muscle power, which represents the combination of strength and speed. Faced with a four-lane intersection, you may have enough strength to walk across the street. But you need power, not just strength, to make that crossing safely before the light changes. Likewise,

Three simple strength and power exercises

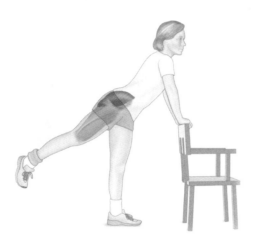 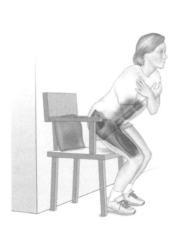 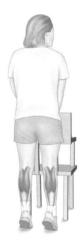

Hip extension

Exercises the muscles of the buttocks and back thighs

Stand 12 inches behind a sturdy chair. Holding on to the back of the chair for balance, bend your trunk forward 45°. Slowly raise your right leg straight out behind you. Lift it as high as possible without bending your knee. Pause. Slowly lower the leg. Do this eight to 12 times. Repeat with your left leg. Rest and repeat on both sides.

Harder variation: Do this move with a small ankle weight. Do the exercise fewer times until you gain strength.

Power move: Lift your leg quickly. Hold briefly. Lower your leg at a normal pace. Do this six to 10 times.

Chair stand

Exercises the muscles of the abdomen, hips, front thighs, and buttocks

Place a sturdy chair so that its back is resting against a wall. Sit at the front of the chair, knees bent, feet flat on the floor and slightly apart. Keeping your back and shoulders straight, stand up slowly, using your hands as little as possible. Slowly sit back down. Do this eight to 12 times. Rest and repeat the entire set.

Power move: Change the move slightly for the last set by rising from the chair quickly. Sit down again at a normal pace.

Standing calf raise

Exercises the calf muscles

Stand with your feet flat on the floor. Hold on to the back of a chair for balance. Raise yourself up on the balls of your feet, as high as possible. Hold briefly, then lower yourself slowly and gently. Do this eight to 12 times. Rest and repeat the set.

Harder variation: Once your balance and strength improve, do one-leg calf raises. Tuck one foot behind the other calf before rising on the ball of your foot; do sets for each leg. Or stand on both feet, but do not hold on to a chair.

Power move: Rise up on the ball of your foot quickly. Hold briefly. Lower yourself at a normal pace.

by helping you react swiftly if you start to trip or lose your balance, power can help prevent falls.

The goal of strength training is to build up your muscles, so you have greater strength and endurance. The goal of power training is to be able to move quickly when needed, such as crossing the street before the light changes. Power training often involves the same exercises you would use for strength training, but with part of the exercise done more quickly. (For examples of how to adapt strength exercises, see "Three simple strength and power exercises," page 28.) Another option is to wear a weighted vest, which adds an extra challenge to power moves. You can also practice power in your daily activities by crossing from one end of the house to the other as fast as you can.

Functional exercises

Functional exercises can help protect or improve mobility. These exercises mimic daily activities—carrying a heavy object across the room, for instance, or squatting to pick up an object from a low shelf. The benefit of these exercises is that they directly target the activities you're likely already doing; the trade-off is that it's more difficult to focus on specific muscle groups and to incrementally build your strength. Functional exercises may be part of a strength training or rehabilitation program, but you can also do your own exercises at home.

Look for activities that challenge you in strength, power, balance, or flexibility, and try to repeat the movement in sets. Use small hand weights or everyday objects like a book or bag of groceries to add a challenge. In this way, you can supplement any exercise routine with small daily activities. One of the best functional exercises is simply walking up and down stairs. If you have the opportunity to take the stairs instead of an escalator or elevator, do it.

A strong core

Exercises that strengthen your body's core are also essential for maintaining mobility and independence. The core isn't just your abdomen; it includes muscles of the back, sides, pelvis, and buttocks. These muscles, which form the central link connecting the upper body and the lower body, are involved in some way in

Strengthening your core

The classic core exercise is a front plank, which exercises and strengthens all your core muscles. But if you have mobility problems, you will probably want to try the modified version below, leaning on a countertop rather than getting down on the floor, as you would in a classic plank.

Front plank on countertop
Wearing nonskid, rubber-soled shoes, stand facing a countertop with your feet together. Tighten your abdominal muscles and lower your upper-body weight onto your forearms on the counter. Clasp your hands together and align your shoulders directly over your elbows. Step back on the balls of your feet until you are balancing your body in a line. Hold for 15 to 60 seconds. Rest and repeat.

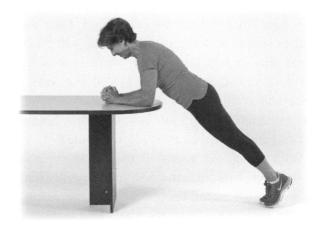

almost everything you do, from carrying a bag of groceries to standing straight or sitting up in a chair. You can move more effortlessly if you're engaging your core muscles and standing up straight, rather than hunching over as you walk. Weakness in the core muscles can lead to back pain, poor posture, and overall frailty, and the effects can spill over into other parts of the body, creating an uneven gait, joint misalignments, balance problems, and a susceptibility to injuries and falls.

Because your core muscles are vital to many kinds of movements, you engage them when you do many types of exercise. But adding some core-focused exercises, like front planks, can help you target core muscles. Unlike sit-ups and crunches, which isolate a few abdominal muscles, planks work all the core muscles at once. If the standard plank is too difficult, try the modified version, leaning against a desk or countertop (see "Strengthening your core," above). ◗

Balancing act

Young, healthy adults may be aware of their sense of balance only when doing something that strongly challenges it, like standing on one leg in a yoga class or jumping from one rock to another while crossing a stream. The fact that most of us don't think much about balance is a testament to how deeply ingrained and instinctive our balance systems are.

In reality, your body is engaged in a constant battle with gravity to keep from falling over. Even something as simple as walking or standing still requires several sensory systems working together to perceive your body's position in space, as well as nerves and muscles to subtly adjust your stance as needed in order to maintain both static balance (while holding a position) and active balance (while moving).

With aging, the acuity of these systems gradually declines. In adulthood and particularly old age, falls and stumbles can bring severe consequences for mobility, such as hip fractures. That's why maintaining balance and avoiding falls is a crucial part of remaining active and mobile.

The body's balance system

Balance is not controlled by a single system in the body. Instead, it is the result of a network of systems working together.

The vestibular system. The key to your sense of balance is the vestibular system in the inner ear (see Figure 8, below). Problems with the vestibular system, such as Ménière's disease (see page 31), can result in vertigo, a sensation of moving or spinning even though you aren't.

The vestibular system has two main components. The first consists of three semicircular canals that are part of what is known as the labyrinth in the inner ear. These canals are ringlike structures that are oriented in different directions, with each one at right angles to the other two. They are filled with a thick fluid that moves as the inner ear tilts. Specialized cells called hair cells sense the movement of this fluid and send signals through the acoustic nerve to the brain. The unique arrangement of the canals means that each is sensitive to different directions of movement; together, they tell

---

Figure 8: The outer, middle, and inner ear

The outer ear consists of the visible parts of the ear: the fleshy outer part (called the auricle), the ear canal, and the eardrum.

The middle ear is an air-filled cavity containing the ossicles, three small bones (malleus, incus, and stapes) that transmit vibrations to the inner ear.

The inner ear is a complex system of membranous canals protected by a bony casing. Inside, the spiral-shaped cochlea contains the hair cells that transmit sound to the auditory nerve, which conducts sound to the brain. **The vestibular system,** which regulates balance, is also part of the inner ear and includes the three semicircular canals, which are the largest part of the labyrinth. The utricle and saccule (not shown) are at the base of the labyrinth.

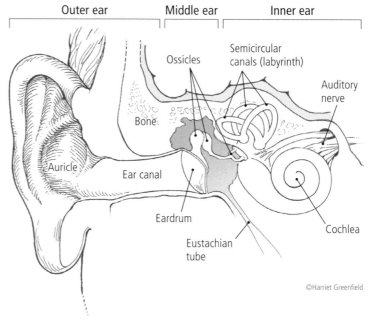

©Harriet Greenfield

Ménière's disease

People with the inner-ear disorder known as Ménière's disease experience severe dizziness and a sensation of spinning (vertigo) that lasts at least 20 minutes, ringing in the ear (tinnitus), hearing loss, and a feeling that there is congestion in the ear. These symptoms typically come and go without warning and can be severely debilitating, interfering with daily life. Loss of balance is a major concern, since that can lead to falls and injury. Hearing loss can become permanent over time.

Ménière's affects about 615,000 people in the United States, and about 45,500 new cases are diagnosed each year. It is most commonly seen in adults between 40 and 60 years old.

Ménière's disease is caused by buildup of endolymph—a thick fluid in the inner ear. In turn, the buildup might be due to a blockage or an anatomic abnormality in the ear, an immune response, infection with a virus, or allergies. There might be a genetic propensity to the disorder, since it's been noted to run in families.

Treating Ménière's disease

You should see an otolaryngologist (ear, nose, and throat doctor) if you think you have Ménière's disease. There's no test for it, but the doctor will ask about your symptoms and perhaps perform a hearing test. Treatments consist of drugs such as the antihistamine meclizine (Antivert, Bonine, Vertin), benzodiazepines (diazepam [Valium], lorazepam [Ativan]), and the scopolamine motion-sickness patch. You will be advised to follow a low-salt diet and prescribed a diuretic to reduce the amount of fluid your body retains and relieve congestion in the ear. You should also try reducing your intake of caffeine, chocolate, and alcohol, and stopping smoking to see if that relieves your symptoms. Finally, your doctor can prescribe the Meniett device to be used three times a day for five minutes each time: an earpiece is placed on the outer ear and intermittently releases pulses of air pressure to displace the endolymph and reduce dizziness.

Injections of the antibiotic gentamicin (Garamycin) can reduce dizziness but may increase the risk of hearing loss. Injections of corticosteroids can also help without risking loss of hearing.

Sixty percent of people will find that Ménière's disease goes away with or without treatment. Surgery to relieve pressure in the inner ear or cut the vestibular nerve is a last-ditch option for severe cases. Alternative treatments like acupuncture and herbal supplements haven't been shown to be of benefit.

---

the brain about the position of the head and any rotational movements it makes through space.

The other part of the vestibular system includes two structures called the utricle and saccule, together known as the otolith organs and also considered to be part of the labyrinth. They are pouches lined with hair cells embedded in a layer of gel, above which is a membrane containing calcium carbonate crystals. When you tilt your head, gravity causes the crystals to move, pulling on the hair cells in the gel below. This relays a signal to the brain letting it know the position and tilt of the head. In addition, the utricle senses horizontal head movements (such as when you're moving forward), and the saccule senses the vertical force of gravity and vertical accelerations (such as when you stand up).

Proprioception and touch. Proprioception is the ability to know where the different parts of your body are in space—whether your legs are straight or bent, whether your arms are down at your sides or over your head, whether you're standing on one leg or lying on your back. It's accomplished through nerves that are distributed throughout the body in muscles, tendons, and joints. Collectively, the information from these nerves informs your brain about what your body is doing, and your brain responds by adjusting your body's position to maintain balance. Added to this internal sense of your body's placement are the external sensations you feel—the pressure of the ground below your feet or your back resting against a chair—which also give you cues about how to position your body.

Vision. Most of us rely on vision to maintain balance. (Try standing on one leg with your eyes closed, and you'll see how much harder it is.) Vision is also important for assessing changes in your surroundings as you move. By looking at the ground ahead of you, for instance, you can anticipate where to place your foot to keep from tripping on a rock or tumbling off a curb. (For more information, see "Vision," page 35.)

Nerves and the spinal cord. Sensory systems collect information about your body and its environment that is transmitted to the brain via the nerves;

nerves also relay your brain's commands back to the body, allowing you to quickly respond to whatever new sensations you're perceiving. Your spinal cord is the information superhighway that channels all this two-way traffic. The spinal cord is also able to initiate reflexes—quick responses to stimuli that don't require the brain's instructions. Reflexes can be important for catching yourself before falling if you're suddenly knocked off balance.

Balance and aging

Keeping your body in balance requires marshaling information from different senses, but the sensory information coming in can diminish with age. That poses a

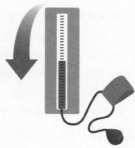
challenge for coordination and balance. Visual acuity—the ability to see objects clearly and in focus—wanes with age, as do night vision, depth perception, and the ability to see contrast between light and dark. Proprioception can also become weaker with age, particularly in people who have damage to the peripheral nerves because of diabetes or another medical condition.

The combination of reduced sensations, declines in muscle strength, and other age-related health problems (see "Blood pressure and fainting," below left) puts people at increasingly greater risk of falling as they age. Falls are the leading cause of death from injury in people over age 65. Each year, one in four people in this age group has a fall.

Falls are the primary cause of broken hips, which pose a serious threat to future mobility. They can also lead to other injuries to the feet, ankles, knees, or back that require a long recovery period. In addition, injuries to the upper body—like the hands, shoulders, or face—can keep you from performing day-to-day tasks independently. Currently, a growing number of older Americans are experiencing fall-related concussions and brain injuries. Even a fall that leads to only minor physical injuries can damage your confidence, making you less likely to exercise and move around on your own.

If you experience a fall or a stumble, take it as an opportunity to assess your health and think about taking steps to improve your balance and coordination. Reduce your risk of falling again by paying more attention to your exercise routine, modifying your home (see "Adapting and fall-proofing your home," page 47), and managing any health conditions that affect balance.

Health conditions that affect balance

In addition to age-related changes, some common health conditions can interfere with balance and coordination, posing challenges for movement—and medications for many conditions can cause similar problems (see "Medications and balance," page 33).

Vestibular disorders. The inner ear structures of the vestibular system can be temporarily or permanently disrupted because of injury, allergies, infec-

© alaroarts | Getty Images

tions, blood circulation problems, or illnesses such as Ménière's disease (see page 31). Vestibular disorders require treatment, which can include balance rehabilitation exercises, medications, and surgery.

Strokes. Strokes are a major cause of mobility loss, and balance can be affected too, through loss of sensation or movement on one side of the body, loss of coordination, weakness, numbness, or vision loss. Strokes can also cause cognitive impairments that make it harder to concentrate, a necessary skill for navigating challenging terrain.

Movement disorders. Parkinson's disease can cause balance-disturbing tremors, rigidity of the legs and torso, slowness of movements, and difficulty coordinating movements.

Peripheral neuropathy. Damage to the peripheral nerves in the arms, legs, feet, and hands can cause tingling, numbness, muscle weakness, or pain that hampers smooth movement. Diabetes is a key cause of this kind of nerve damage. It can also result from injury, alcoholism, or infection.

Excess weight. Overweight and obesity can throw off balance and make you more prone to falling. People who are obese are also more likely to become disabled after a fall.

Reducing the risk of falls

The first step toward keeping yourself or a loved one from falling is to know when there's a problem. Look for these warning signs:

- difficulty climbing stairs without leaning on a rail
- fatigue when performing basic tasks like housework
- leaning on furniture to cross a room
- hesitancy walking and negotiating steps and uneven surfaces
- requiring more assistance getting in and out of chairs, a car, or a shower or bath
- changes in gait—for example, excessive slowness, favoring one side over another, or shuffling
- fear of falling (people who are afraid of falls become increasingly hesitant and sedentary, which weakens their bodies and puts them at further risk)
- avoiding bathing, changing clothes, or other basic tasks, because of fear of falls or injuries.

▶ **Medications and balance**

A long list of medications can affect balance and raise the risk of falling, mostly because of their potential to cause side effects like dizziness, drowsiness, confusion, or fainting. As people get older they tend to take multiple medications, which can cause a greater number or intensity of side effects; taking four or more medications at once is associated with a higher risk of falling. Some types of drugs that can cause problems are

- psychiatric drugs such as antipsychotics, tricyclic antidepressants, and anti-anxiety drugs
- anticholinergic/antispasmodic drugs
- muscle relaxants
- antihistamines
- pain medications such as opioids and nonsteroidal anti-inflammatory drugs (NSAIDs)
- heart drugs, such as anti-arrhythmics, vasodilators, and digoxin.

Not all of these will cause problems for all people. Alert your doctor to any side effects you feel that could put you at risk of falls or injuries. Your doctor can help you weigh the risks of the medication or adopt strategies to manage the side effects.

If you notice any of these, a conversation with a doctor is in order. A physical therapist or another clinician can create a program to reduce your fall risk. This includes exercises to build strength, improve your gait and sense of balance, increase your activity level, and build your confidence. Several evidence-based fall prevention programs have been shown to help reduce the risk of falling. They range from one-time workshops to multiweek exercise programs; some are based on the slow, controlled movements of tai chi. The National Council on Aging has resources, including a list of evidence-based programs for fall prevention at www.ncoa.org/older-adults/health/prevention/falls-prevention.

You also may need to make small shifts in your day-to-day behavior, like moving more slowly in low-lit places and pausing to get your bearings after standing and before walking. Some clinical programs also include a home visit to assess whether you can make changes to your home to help prevent falls (see "Adapting and fall-proofing your home," see page 47).

Balance exercises

Muscles and bones need to be challenged or else they deteriorate. The same is true of balance. Fortunately, balance and coordination can be maintained with practice and even improve over time.

Many types of physical activity challenge the balance system. If you do yoga, dance, or tai chi, you're giving your balance system a workout by putting your body in challenging positions. However, if most of your exercise is using a stationary bike or weight machines, or simply walking on a path, you may be missing out on a chance to build up your balance abilities along with your strength and cardiovascular fitness. Here are two targeted exercises you can do at home to challenge and improve your balance.

Heel-to-toe walk ▶
Position your heel just in front of the toes of the opposite foot as you walk forward for eight to 12 steps. Heel and toes should actually touch each time you take a step. If necessary, steady yourself by putting one hand on a counter as you walk at first, and then work toward doing this without support. Repeat two to four times.

Single-leg stance ▼
Stand on one foot for up to 30 seconds. Put your foot down and repeat on the opposite side. Perform two to four times on each leg. If this is too hard, steady yourself by holding on to the back of a chair at first, then work toward doing this without support. For an added challenge, you can add ankle weights.

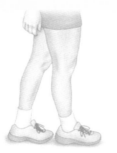
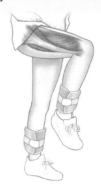

Overcoming the fear of falling

Fear can be a helpful signal; it can bring your attention to problems—such as a balance disorder, reduced vision, or muscle weakness—that keep you from moving confidently. But fear can also undermine you. Persistent worrying about a fall, if it's unwarranted, may cause you to limit your mobility unnecessarily and avoid routine daily activities. It's estimated that half of older adults are concerned enough about potential falls that they have begun to restrict or avoid activities that would be beneficial for their health.

How can you build your confidence? If you don't trust yourself when walking, it's important to talk with your doctor to understand the cause of the fear. Is it a sign of a health problem—perhaps a vision problem or arthritis pain—that you need to address? Do you need a hip replacement or a new pair of glasses? Or are you worried about your sense of balance?

Exercise is essential for helping to maintain strength in your legs, buttocks, and core, all of which are important for balance. Certain types of exercise, such as Pilates, yoga, and tai chi, are particularly helpful for balance. (Harvard Medical School offers Special Health Reports that cover most of these types of exercise, including *Better Balance, Gentle Core Exercises, An Introduction to Yoga,* and *An Introduction to Tai Chi;* see "Resources," page 53, for ordering information.) Adopting such a program can help build your confidence—and prevent devastating falls.

If you've already had a fall, think about building confidence back gradually as you recover. Depending on how badly you've been injured, you may need to work with a physical therapist to regain your strength and range of motion. One type of therapy you can do with a physical therapist is called gait training. In this therapy, you work not just on strengthening muscles, but also improving posture and developing good walking form, so that you move more fluidly. Once people recover 90% of their normal strength, they start to regain their confidence. If you've been prescribed a cane or a walker, don't hesitate to rely on it for balance and support. If strong relatives can accompany you on walks, so much the better. Stick to walking in familiar places that you know well, and don't try to go farther than you normally would. Avoid walking at night or in wet or icy conditions. If you're afraid of falling, try exercises that don't carry that risk, like swimming or pool aerobics, in which the water supports you. ▼

The mind and senses: Staying sharp

Mobility requires more than just bones, muscles, tendons, and cartilage. It requires being able to assess your environment so you can move through it safely and effectively. To get from point A to point B, you must know where point B is, whether there are any steps or rough terrain between them, and what movements you need to accomplish to reach your goal. And that's just walking; you need a whole different set of skills to operate a car. When driving, you need to sense and respond to fast-moving traffic and navigate complex routes. If you're moving through your own neighborhood or city, you must access your memories of the streets, and if you're driving in unfamiliar places, you must locate and respond to street signs and other directional cues (see "Driving: Staying up to the challenge," page 36).

Vision

Humans are visual animals. Although people who are visually impaired or even completely blind can learn to move around adeptly by using other senses, the rest of us rely heavily on our vision for day-to-day tasks, and vision is the sense that most people are most afraid of losing. Age-related vision loss can dramatically limit your daily activities and can make living with other health conditions even more challenging. Yet many people do not think about the health of their eyes or seek out medical attention for vision problems until the problem is severe.

The visual system undergoes many changes with age. In particular, the lens inside the eye grows harder, which can cause presbyopia, an inability to clearly distinguish close objects, such as the printed words of a book. Even changes that seem cosmetic can affect vision; muscles in the face shrink, while skin gets thinner and begins to sag—and sagging eyelids and weakening muscles can interfere with normal vision.

While such changes are part of normal aging,

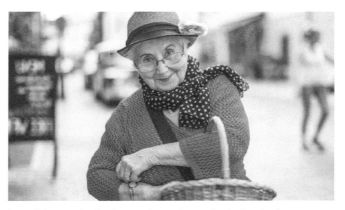

It can't be emphasized enough: staying active is the single most important thing you can do to maintain mobility and independence, no matter your age or health status.

others could signal a vision-related disease. The following conditions are the most common causes of vision impairment.

Cataracts. The lens of the eye can become cloudy over time, a condition known as a cataract. Cataracts are extremely common; most people over age 60 have some cloudiness of the lens, and about half of people ages 65 to 74 and 70% of those 75 and older have cataracts. Cataracts develop slowly, so you may not realize you're experiencing symptoms at first. Objects may look slightly blurry or dim, and your eyes may be sensitive to the glare of bright lights. You may become more nearsighted or begin to notice a lessening in your ability to see colors and to see at night.

Age is the biggest risk factor, but you're more likely to get cataracts if you have a family history of cataracts or if you smoke, drink alcohol excessively, have had an eye injury, use corticosteroid medications, have diabetes, are obese, or have spent considerable time in the sun without proper eyewear and hats to provide protection (see "Choosing sunglasses," page 37).

At the early stage of cataracts, be proactive about aiding your vision. Change your eyeglass or contact prescription if needed, keep your house or workspace

Continued on page 37

© Eva-Katalin | Getty Images

Driving: Staying up to the challenge

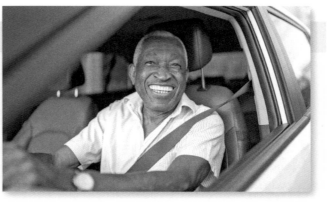

© FG Trade I Getty Images

For many people, driving a car is a key part of maintaining independence, particularly if they live in places without easy public transportation. If you're one of them, will you be able to keep driving—and if so, for how long? Driving requires coordination of the senses, brain, and body. But health problems and common age-related changes can affect your ability to drive safely; even subtle changes can affect your reaction time. Following are some of the issues that can arise, along with possible solutions that might keep you driving for a while longer.

But it's also important to recognize when driving is no longer safe for you. Fortunately, the increasing availability of options such as volunteer driver programs, para-transit services, Uber, and Lyft has made it easier to get around efficiently and independently without sitting behind the wheel.

Sensory changes

The most obvious driving-related change is vision problems that make it difficult to read distant traffic signs or nearby dashboard indicators, see at night, spot objects in your peripheral vision, or cope with glare from oncoming headlights or sunlight reflecting off cars ahead of you. Hearing loss can also affect your driving skills, by keeping you from noticing outside noise such as sirens and horns.

Solutions: If you wear glasses or contact lenses, use them when you drive and keep your prescription up to date. Loss of night vision can't be corrected with glasses, but an anti-glare coating on your eyeglasses can reduce the temporary blindness caused by oncoming headlights. Consider installing wider side- and rearview mirrors to give better visibility, and make sure your dashboard lights are at their brightest setting. Schedule regular eye exams to catch any age-related eye conditions that can impair vision. Keep noise inside the car to a minimum, and cut back on night driving.

Chronic conditions

Chronic physical challenges—such as arthritis pain, the tremors of Parkinson's disease, or the pain of chronic back problems—may make it difficult to grip a steering wheel, turn to look for traffic, or press the brakes. If you have diabetes, driving skills can become impaired when blood sugar levels drop too low, causing blurry vision, confusion, and even loss of consciousness.

Solutions: Manage your condition with help from your doctor. Keep active by exercising and stretching, which can help maintain the flexibility and strength you need to operate a car. If you use insulin to treat your diabetes and have had episodes of low blood sugar, check your blood sugar level before you drive, and keep a blood glucose meter in the car, as well as a quick-acting source of glucose such as juice.

Cognitive changes

In general, mental sharpness fades as you age, which can slow your reaction time—for example, when a child runs into the street or a car cuts in front of you. Mild cognitive impairment and dementia can cause drivers to get lost, become confused in high-traffic areas, and misjudge distance and timing, which are crucial to driving.

Solutions: As much as possible, avoid driving in challenging conditions, such as during rush hour, in high-traffic areas, along unfamiliar routes, at night, or in bad weather conditions. Avoid mental distractions by putting cellphones and other electronic devices away; making calls and sending texts or emails while driving can impair drivers as much as drinking does—and can be illegal, depending on your state.

Medications and alcohol

Medications may cause side effects such as confusion, dizziness, and drowsiness. Alcohol impairs driving at any age, but when you are older, you metabolize alcohol differently, especially if you are taking certain medications.

Solutions: Ask your pharmacist to evaluate all of your drugs and supplements for their potential impact on your driving skills. Never drink and drive, and be aware that you may need to allow more time for alcohol to leave your system as you age.

Other considerations

To help you stay on top of your driving skills, think about taking one of the drivers' safety courses offered for older drivers by either AARP (www.aarp.org/auto/driver-safety) or AAA (www.seniordriving.aaa.com). These courses cover everything from loss of vision, hearing, cognitive function, and motor function to the side effects of common medications.

At some point, though, older people need to make tough decisions about whether to stop driving. Based on current life expectancies, most older drivers will outlive their ability to drive safely by several years. An occupational therapist can perform a comprehensive driving assessment to determine whether you can continue to drive safely, and may recommend modifications, restrictions, or rehabilitation and training to cope with challenges to driving. Or he or she might conclude that, unfortunately, you can no longer drive safely.

Continued from page 35

well lit, and make sure your computer monitor is positioned so that there isn't glare from overhead lights or windows (you can also install an anti-glare screen on your monitor). Use eyeglasses with an antireflective coating on the lenses.

The only proven treatment for cataracts is lens replacement surgery (see Figure 9, page 38). This involves taking out the cloudy lens in your eye and replacing it with a clear artificial lens, called an intraocular lens. It is an extremely common and safe procedure; it can now be performed on an outpatient basis under local anesthesia, without a hospital stay. Some people never need it, while others can safely delay it for months or years, or have surgery in one eye but not the other. But while avoiding an invasive procedure is appealing, it's important not to delay or avoid surgery if you're having vision problems that interfere with your daily activities, inhibit your independence, or threaten your safety.

Glaucoma. Glaucoma is a condition that damages the optic nerve, which relays information from the eye's retina to the brain. This damage can result in vision loss or blindness. Although it can occur in anyone, it's more common in people over 60, African Americans, Mexican Americans, and Asians, and people with a family history of glaucoma. Other conditions—such as diabetes, high blood pressure, and severe nearsightedness or farsightedness—can also increase the risk of developing glaucoma.

The most common type of the disease, called open-angle glaucoma, is caused by poor drainage of aqueous humor (the fluid in the front of the eye), leading to a backup of the fluid and a gradual but persistent elevation of pressure inside the eye. Eventually, this pressure cuts off blood vessels and kills nerve cells, beginning with tiny nerve fibers affecting peripheral vision but gradually closing in until central vision is lost as well. However, other factors in addition to high intraocular pressure also seem to play a role in promoting the death of nerve cells, since not everyone with high pressure in the eye gets glaucoma, and research shows that not everyone with glaucoma has high pressure.

By the time you begin to notice visual disturbances (often poor peripheral vision, blind spots, or difficulty

▶ Choosing sunglasses

A good way to protect your vision is to wear sunglasses that help block ultraviolet (UV) rays of the sun. In addition to its well-known effects on skin, UV light can cause growths on the eye surface and boost the risk of developing cataracts and macular degeneration.

Wearing sunglasses also makes vision more comfortable by reducing visible light, making it easier for you to navigate a sunny environment. Look for glasses that are labeled as blocking at least 99% of two different kinds of ultraviolet rays, UVA and UVB. Or choose glasses labeled "UV400," which block all UVA and UVB radiation and other potentially harmful rays. Polarized lenses don't block UV rays, but they can reduce glare from reflective light when you're driving or spending time on the water.

Another consideration is the shape of the lenses. Glasses that are larger and wrap around the eyes offer more protection than small lenses that allow a lot of light through the sides of the glasses. Wearing a hat is also important to reduce the amount of sun that your glasses have to block.

All people should protect their eyes from UV rays, but it's especially important for people who already have eye disease or have had cataract surgery. In addition, certain antibiotics and other drugs, like amiodarone (Cordarone), make the eyes more sensitive to light, so people who take these medications should be especially vigilant about wearing sunglasses.

adjusting to the dark), the disease has already become severe. A doctor can detect glaucoma before you notice it, which makes regular check-ups important. For open-angle glaucoma, treatment usually begins with topical medications—eye drops or sometimes ointments—administered once or more a day. Depending on the severity of the condition, multiple drops and sometimes pills may be required. Most ophthalmologists begin with the lowest effective dose to minimize cost and potential side effects. Should medicines fail to control pressure, surgery may be necessary.

Age-related macular degeneration. Age-related macular degeneration (AMD) is another slowly progressing disease. It affects one of the most important places in the eye for vision—the macula, a bundle of cells at the center of the retina responsible for sharp

Figure 9: Lens replacement surgery for cataracts

1.

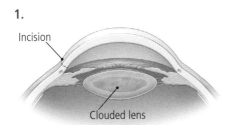

The ophthalmologist makes a small incision about an eighth of an inch long in the side of the cornea.

2.

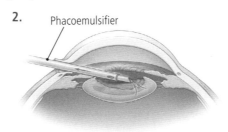

Using a small, needle-like probe called a phacoemulsifier, the doctor directs high-frequency sound waves through the lens to break it into small pieces, which are then gently suctioned out through the probe.

3.

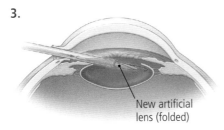

The artificial lens, which is folded to fit inside the probe, is inserted through the same incision.

4.

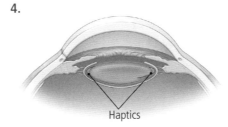

The new lens unfolds inside the lens capsule and is held in place by tiny loops called haptics.

central vision. There are two forms of the condition:

- Dry AMD, the more common form, is caused by thinning of the retina and loss of cells that detect light.
- Wet AMD is less common but more serious. It occurs when abnormal blood vessels grow into the retina and cause a marked loss of central vision.

AMD is most common in people over 60, though it can occur earlier. As in glaucoma, symptoms often appear late in the disease process, but the vision loss is different. You may notice a blurred spot in the center of your vision that can progress to blank spots; also, sometimes objects appear less bright. AMD does not cause total blindness, but at later stages it can hamper your mobility and independence by making it difficult to drive, read, use computers or smartphones, or do work and activities that involve seeing things up close.

Although age is the biggest risk factor for AMD, smoking more than doubles your risk; Caucasians and people with a family history of AMD are also at higher

risk of developing the disease. The only current treatment for dry AMD is a diet that includes leafy green vegetables—combined with dietary supplementation with a combination of antioxidants called the AREDS2 formulation (after the second Age-Related Eye Disease Study, which tested it). Laser therapy is being investigated and has been shown to be effective in some cases; repeat treatments appear to be necessary, however. Wet AMD is treated with injections of anti-vascular endothelial growth factor (VEGF) drugs, which inhibit the growth of new blood vessels in the eye.

Diabetic or hypertensive retinopathy. High blood sugar (the hallmark of diabetes) and high blood pressure both damage small blood vessels in the retina. Over time, this leads to vision loss and blindness. Although there is no cure for either condition, treatments for diabetic retinopathy include laser therapies, anti-VEGF medications, and a surgical procedure called vitrectomy to slow the damage and prevent blindness. Drugs to reduce blood pressure are prescribed to manage hypertensive retinopathy. Working to control blood sugar and blood pressure can keep vision loss at bay. Having yearly eye exams that include a retina check is also important.

Living with vision problems

The most important step to living successfully with vision problems is recognizing them. Too often, people either ignore or deny changes to their vision. That can keep them from adapting successfully and, if the vision loss is severe, can put themselves or others in harm's way. Taking steps to stay active and connected in spite of low vision will ensure that the rest of your health doesn't suffer.

An ophthalmologist, optometrist, or rehabilitation specialist can help you develop strategies to cope with low vision. Focus on what could be changed in your daily environment to make it easier for you to see important objects. One strategy is to create contrasts—make sure that stairs, doors, or objects you need to find stand out from their surroundings, either with bright colors or differences in shade. You'll see white pills better if you place them on a dark tablecloth, and placing brightly colored tape on stairs, door handles, and appliances can help you distinguish them. You may need brighter lights than before, particularly when reading.

Many devices and products are available to help. Magnifying lenses, either incorporated into eyeglass lenses, held in the hand, or mounted on a stand, can help you do close work like reading or sewing. Magnifying mirrors can help with shaving or applying cosmetics. An e-reader, such as a Kindle, allows you to adjust the size of the type, and many software programs and apps will also enlarge text on a screen. There are even text-to-speech programs that can read text on a screen aloud to you. No single product can compensate for low vision. Instead, try different task-specific tools to accomplish the activities that matter to you. The key is to have patience with yourself. Learning to use magnifying lenses and other aids is like learning to walk with crutches—it may require some effort and adjustment, but will help you maintain your everyday activities.

Preserving eye health

Vision changes and eye diseases are common consequences of aging, but they're not inevitable. It's estimated that as much as 8% of all blindness could be avoided with proper treatment and preventive measures.

The most important step toward keeping eyes healthy is to get regular dilated eye exams, particularly if you have a personal or family history of eye disease. People who have had longstanding vision problems and require glasses and contacts usually have regular exams when they update their prescriptions, but other people may fail to think about their eye health. The American Academy of Ophthalmologists recommends an eye exam every two years for people at any age at high risk of eye disease, as well as everyone over age 65. But get any vision problems checked right away, and keep glasses or contact lenses updated with a current prescription.

Quitting or avoiding smoking is another important step to preserving eye health. Following a healthy lifestyle and managing chronic diseases such as diabetes and high blood pressure will ultimately benefit your vision. Diet also plays a role in eye health: diets rich in leafy green vegetables like collard greens, kale, and spinach, and fish high in omega-3 fatty acids, help protect vision.

Another way to safeguard your vision is to wear sunglasses when needed to protect your eyes from ultraviolet rays (see "Choosing sunglasses," page 37).

Hearing

If you've noticed problems with your hearing, you're not alone. About one-third of people in their 60s and half of those over 75 have some level of hearing loss. It's estimated that some 29 million Americans could benefit from a hearing aid. Men tend to lose their hearing earlier than women and have more severe hearing loss. Some hearing loss is related to a physical obstruction of the ear canal by earwax, debris, inflammation, or fluid. But most hearing loss is caused by damage to the sensory hair cells in the ear or the nerves that transmit auditory signals to the brain.

Presbycusis, or age-related hearing loss, is the leading cause of hearing problems. Besides age, other factors that contribute to hearing loss are exposure to loud noise, smoking, various diseases, and exposure to some medications or chemicals.

It may not be obvious that hearing loss can harm independence, since we use our eyes to get around much more than we use our ears. But recent research has shown that preventing and treating hearing loss not only preserves and restores your hearing, but also protects your brain from decline and possibly even from dementia. The reasons for this association are not yet known. One possibility is that when people struggle with their hearing, they often withdraw from social interactions with family and friends, which leads to depression. This isolation in itself is a known risk factor for dementia. Another possibility is that hearing loss accelerates a decline in brain function that affects other processes such as perception and cognition.

Treating hearing loss

Age-related hearing loss is often a gradual process, and you may adjust to incremental changes without noticing them—in fact, only 20% of people over 65 with hearing loss that is moderate to profound recognize that they have a hearing problem. People often lose the ability to hear some frequencies of sound rather than all sounds. It's common to first find it difficult to hear high-frequency sounds like a hiss or whisper, or sounds like "s" and "th" and "f" in speech. You may have trouble hearing certain sounds at low volumes, notice a lack of clarity, or feel you can hear the words people say but can't understand them. The problem is usually most obvious in situations with background noise, like when you're trying to have a conversation at a restaurant or you're watching TV with a fan running in the background.

Age-related hearing loss does not necessarily require treatment, but it's still important to have your hearing tested by an audiologist if you suspect you're not hearing as well as you used to, and to have any hearing loss monitored. It may result from a treatable condition like wax or fluid buildup. If the hearing loss is mild, an audiologist can recommend strategies to keep it from interfering with conversations or activities.

If your hearing loss is serious enough to require a hearing aid, the good news is that technological advances have made hearing aids smaller, more discreet, and better with less distortion. There are many choices in the size and shape of the hearing aids, as well as features like reducing background noise, amplifying selective sounds, and connecting wirelessly via Bluetooth to a cellphone. Talk to your audiologist about what type of hearing aid is best suited to your hearing loss, lifestyle, and budget, as well as about assistive listening devices such as phone-amplifying devices, apps, and closed-circuit systems, which are available at places of worship, theaters, and auditoriums.

Preventing hearing loss

To prevent hearing loss, turn down the volume. Loud noise can destroy specialized cells in the ears that sense sound. It's not just rock concerts that hurt hearing; leaf and snow blowers, lawn mowers, chain saws, wood chippers, and even loud appliances in the home (like hair dryers) can cause damage. Use earplugs or earmuffs if you're going to be hearing loud noises. If you listen to music on headphones or earbuds, be aware that safe listening depends on both the volume and the length of time you're listening. Keep the volume low, and don't turn it up to drown out background noise (invest in noise-canceling headphones instead). A good rule is to limit listening time to an hour a day.

Mobility and your brain

The brain is the master controller of movement, so it's not surprising that changes in brain function can cause problems with mobility. Taking care of your brain is part and parcel of staying mobile as you age, as well as avoiding further declines in physical health if you're living with a chronic condition. Mobility is linked to a few different brain functions.

Attention. Almost every mental task involves some degree of attention—focusing on one object or aspect of your environment and not others. Older adults sometimes have difficulty dividing and switching their attention (though they are generally better at sustaining attention on a single task compared with younger adults). This can make it hard to accomplish tasks that put complex demands on the brain and senses, like navigating a crowded airport or driving a car. Declines in attention are linked to gait changes and susceptibility to injuries and falls.

Executive function. The ability to make plans, organize your schedule and life, manage your time, behave and speak appropriately, and adapt your behavior based on past experiences is part of a set of skills often referred to collectively as "executive function." As the name implies, these are high-level skills that help you control your life and manage social situations—think of them as your ability to be your own boss. Declines in executive function are linked to mobility problems and falls.

Working memory. Working memory is the ability to hold information you just learned in your mind for a short time and manipulating that information—for example, calculating a tip on a restaurant bill. Loss of

▶ Gait and cognition

Doctors used to consider physical abilities separately from mental abilities when they evaluated older patients. But increasingly, there's been a realization that how you walk (which tells a doctor about your physical health and risk of falls) changes when there is a decline in how well your brain accomplishes certain tasks.

It's long been appreciated that people with dementia have a greater risk of falls. And falls can be particularly devastating to this population; people who have cognitive problems are five times more likely to require institutional care than people who fall but are in good cognitive health. Interventions designed to prevent falls (using balance training and other techniques) have had less success in people with dementia.

working memory has been linked to a slower gait in older adults and may reflect a general difficulty devoting brain power to complex tasks (see "Gait and cognition," above).

Mood and motivation. Anything that reduces your motivation to get out and about, from a stroke-related brain injury to depression, can affect how motivated you are to be active, take on physical challenges, and cope with health problems (see "Mind, mood, and mobility," page 5).

Keeping your brain healthy

Science still has much to learn about the aging brain and how to ward off mental decline. But the following actions have consistently been linked to better brain functioning with age.

Stay physically active. Exercise can improve mental function in people with mild declines in thinking skills and memory.

Manage medical conditions. High blood pressure, high cholesterol, obesity, diabetes, hearing loss, and hormonal changes can lead to declines in thinking skills and memory. By keeping these conditions under control, you can help avoid the negative feedback loop between poor physical health, mental decline, and diminished mobility.

Check your medications. Many medications have side effects that can cloud the brain, including prescription medications to treat depression, overactive bladder, and heartburn. Even common over-the-counter drugs for allergies and colds can make you feel sleepy and confused. Many people take multiple medications, which can cause side effects to be more pronounced than from one drug alone.

Exercise your brain. Mental challenges can help keep the brain healthy and contribute to overall health. For you, that might involve reading, taking classes, writing in a journal, doing crossword puzzles, playing chess, participating in a book club or discussion group, taking on a volunteer position, using a computer, or mastering a new hobby or craft. The most effective strategies are those that require learning new skills or information, such as studying a foreign language or taking up a musical instrument. Whatever activities you choose, look for ways to engage mentally with new ideas, situations, or skills. And the more the better: a study published in *Neurology* in 2019 found that engaging in two or more stimulating activities in later life reduced the risk of developing mild cognitive dysfunction. More formal "brain training," such as computer games designed to challenge memory, processing speed, or reasoning, may also help, but they mainly improve your ability to perform the specific task in the game, and most of the studies on them are short-term. More research is needed to see if these programs can actually slow or prevent age-related cognitive decline.

Get enough rest. Lack of sleep can cause confusion, forgetfulness, and fatigue. It has also been linked to weight gain, lowered immunity, and depression. Older people have more sleep-related problems, including insomnia and obstructive sleep apnea (briefly stopping breathing repeatedly during the night). More recent studies have reported a link between dementia and sleep deprivation and emphasized the importance of making restful sleep part of a healthy daily routine.

Stay social. Connections with others—whether they are family members, friends, neighbors, or people with a shared hobby—can help improve mental performance in older people. Social connections can also provide a buffer against the damaging effects of stress, depression, and anxiety. ♥

How weight and diet can sabotage your mobility

Many people lose mobility because of their weight. Excess weight—especially when it tips the scales into the obese range—can impair mobility by making it difficult to rise from a chair, walk around the block, or climb stairs. It can rob you of energy, making simple day-to-day tasks exhausting. And it's a risk factor for several chronic health problems that can affect mobility, such as cardiovascular disease, type 2 diabetes, and osteoarthritis. What's more, if you already have osteoarthritis, excess weight can accelerate the course of the disease, producing greater pain—and greater disincentive to move. While it's possible to be both overweight and physically fit, it's more common be out of shape and lack muscle strength. Eventually, excess weight, inactivity, weakness, and weight-related health problems tend to feed into one another, leading to a loss of mobility and independence.

If you are already experiencing problems with mobility and independence, it may be very difficult for you to lose weight. But weight management is still important, so that you don't continue to put on pounds. Exercise, as recommended in this report, will help you avoid weight gain. But your diet is also crucial to managing your weight, whether you're trying to stay at your current weight or lose some.

Moreover, your diet affects your ability to move and stay healthy in other ways beyond weight. Your body depends on the nutrients in food to build bones, power muscle, repair and replace tissues, and keep your brain active and your heart pumping. Epidemiological studies on older adults have linked low fruit and vegetable intake with higher risks of disability, and low levels of certain nutrients are linked with higher rates of frailty. So a healthy diet, weight control, and physical fitness work together to help keep your body strong and free of disease.

While weighing too much is an increasingly common problem among older adults, weighing too little can also be a cause for concern. Many older adults find that their appetite gradually declines over time. Eating too little can contribute to frailty, ill health, and undernourishment. Making good choices about what you eat can help you have energy throughout the day and stay healthy for a long time.

Managing weight effectively

Controlling your weight is important at every age. And the most successful way to do that is through a combination of diet and physical activity. If you have problems with mobility, exercise becomes a challenge. But the Physical Activity Guidelines for Americans from the U.S. Department of Health and

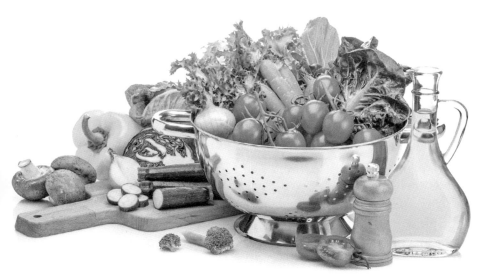

While your requirement for calories declines with age, the need for key nutrients does not. That means that it's important to keep eating nutrient-dense foods like vegetables.

Human Services emphasize that everyone—even older adults and people with disabilities—should try to meet the goal of at least 150 minutes a week of moderate aerobic activity, with some activity every day. Tennis and jogging may be out of the question, but there is still a lot you can do. Many senior centers offer chair aerobics, for example. Another option is to purchase an inexpensive minicycle that you can place in front of your armchair, so that you can pedal while you watch TV.

If possible, add some strength training to your routine (see "Building a strength training routine," page 27). Not only will this help with balance and everyday activities, but the added muscle you build will also rev up your metabolism, since muscles burn calories for fuel, while fat cells mainly store calories.

If you have a temporary health setback or develop a chronic con-dition like arthritis, work with your doctor or physical therapist to find an exercise routine you can manage; many people gain weight during illness and recovery and find it hard to take the weight off.

When it comes to weight management, however, diet is even more important than exercise. Think of it this way: for an average 150-pound person, it takes an hour of walking at 3 mph to burn 250 calories. It's easier to cut out a 20-ounce bottle of sugary soda (240 calories).

Unfortunately, your metabolism gradually slows with age, so the body requires fewer calories each day. Many people find it hard to cut back on the amount of food they eat, and they begin to gain weight. The same challenge faces people who have become less active because of disease, lost mobility, or disability. But while your requirement for calories declines, the need for important nutrients like pro-tein, vitamins, and minerals stays the same. That means as you get older, it's even more important to make each meal count by choosing healthy, nutrient-rich foods rather than those full of "empty" calories.

There are some strategies you can use to help you eat less. For example, you can trick your mind by buying smaller plates, so portions seem larger, and by rearranging your cupboards, so snack foods are out of sight (see "Strategies to outwit your appetite," page 45). But the most important thing for both weight loss and general health is to concentrate on foods that are nutrient-dense but low in calories, such as fruits, vegetables, and beans.

Keys to a healthy diet

Aging and the loss of mobility can make it challenging to maintain a healthy diet. You may find it harder to cook or go grocery shopping if you're struggling with arthritis pain, for instance. Grief following the death of a spouse can also make you lose motivation to cook and to eat on a regular schedule. But maintaining a healthy diet doesn't need to be complex or burdensome. You can break it down into a few basic steps:

- Choose mostly plant-based foods that are unprocessed or minimally processed.
- Strive to eat a variety of fruits, vegetables, and whole grains over the course of the week, in order to ensure a balance of important nutrients.

- Eat only as much as you need, keeping your calorie intake and physical activity level in balance.

Choosing unprocessed or minimally processed foods is especially important. An apple, for instance, contains fiber, vitamins, minerals, and other nutrients called phytochemicals or phytonutrients, which play important roles in health. Process that apple into apple juice, and you lose fiber and some of those other nutrients. Turn the apple into a packaged fruit snack, and you get mostly sugar.

The same goes for grains. Bread made entirely from whole grains is far better than bread made from refined flour—which is missing the fiber-rich outer casing (the bran) and the nutrient-rich inner germ of each kernel. (Even if refined grain is "fortified," manufacturers have added only a limited range of nutrients back in.) Whole, unprocessed grains—such as quinoa or barley—are even better since they lack the added sugar and salt that bread usually has.

And there's another problem with processed foods, in addition to the loss of fiber and other nutrients. Processed foods often contain extra sugar, fat, and salt to make them tastier.

Processed foods are often a major part of the diet of older adults and people with mobility limitations because they are convenient, easy to store and eat, and longer-lasting compared with fresh fruits and vegetables. But unprocessed or minimally processed foods can also be convenient: frozen fruits and vegetables, canned salmon, low-sodium canned beans, unsalted nuts, and prepackaged carrot sticks are all examples of healthy foods that are easy to store and use. If mobility problems make it difficult for you to shop for fresh foods, you can seek out grocery- or meal-delivery services to help you keep fresh foods in the house. If you are losing teeth or have trouble chewing, try pureeing fruits and vegetables into smoothies. That way you can get all the benefits of the nutrients in an easy-to-swallow food.

To help people make healthy food choices, nutrition experts from Harvard Medical School and the Harvard T.H. Chan School of Public Health devised the Healthy Eating Plate (see Figure 10, at left). The Healthy Eating Plate gives a detailed, evidence-based model that can help you plan which foods should have a more prominent place in your diet, which ones you should avoid, and how to think about balancing foods in your diet for your overall health.

Fill half your plate with fruits and vegetables. Fruits and vegetables are high in important nutrients, but (for the most part) low in calories, so they are an important part of your strategy. *Simple tips:* Add some frozen vegetables to low-sodium soup stock for a quick, healthy soup. Keep a bowl of fruit handy and make a habit of eating a piece of fruit after a meal.

Figure 10: Harvard's Healthy Eating Plate

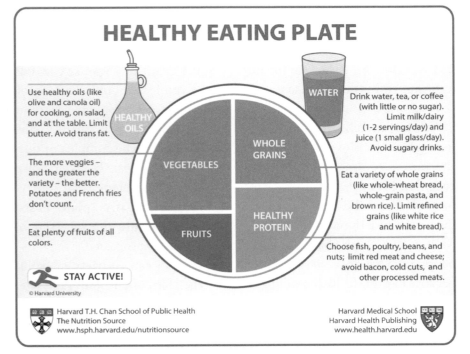

HEALTHY EATING PLATE

Use healthy oils (like olive and canola oil) for cooking, on salad, and at the table. Limit butter. Avoid trans fat.

The more veggies – and the greater the variety – the better. Potatoes and French fries don't count.

Eat plenty of fruits of all colors.

WATER — Drink water, tea, or coffee (with little or no sugar). Limit milk/dairy (1-2 servings/day) and juice (1 small glass/day). Avoid sugary drinks.

Eat a variety of whole grains (like whole-wheat bread, whole-grain pasta, and brown rice). Limit refined grains (like white rice and white bread).

Choose fish, poultry, beans, and nuts; limit red meat and cheese; avoid bacon, cold cuts, and other processed meats.

HEALTHY OILS / VEGETABLES / WHOLE GRAINS / FRUITS / HEALTHY PROTEIN

STAY ACTIVE!
© Harvard University

Harvard T.H. Chan School of Public Health
The Nutrition Source
www.hsph.harvard.edu/nutritionsource

Harvard Medical School
Harvard Health Publishing
www.health.harvard.edu

Make a quarter of your plate whole grains. Not only are whole grains more nutritious, but choosing whole grains over refined grains can also help curb your appetite. *Simple tips:* Cook a large batch of quinoa or another whole grain and use it as a side dish or on top of salads throughout the week.

Fill the remaining quarter of your plate with healthy protein. The final quarter of the plate holds healthy protein like fish, beans, soy products, nuts, seeds, or poultry. Protein is particularly important for maintaining muscle strength with age. Although most Americans get more than enough protein in their diet, many older adults don't. Eating lots of protein won't by itself keep your muscles strong—for that, you need to exercise. But without enough protein, your body can't replace or build muscle tissue. It's a good idea to eat some protein with every meal or snack. *Simple tips:* Add some low-sodium canned beans or a hard-boiled egg to a salad, toss chopped nuts or seeds onto your cereal at breakfast, slather some peanut butter on an apple, pair nuts with carrot slices, or have a cup of plain low-fat or nonfat Greek yogurt with fruit.

Stay hydrated. Dehydration can affect your energy level and cause constipation, headaches, and dizziness, which can lead to mobility-impairing falls. Choose low- or no-calorie liquids like water or seltzer, coffee, and tea, and avoid

sugary drinks. *Simple tips:* Beverages aren't the only way to hydrate. You get quite a lot of water from the foods you eat, such as fruits (like watermelon or strawberries), vegetables (like cucumbers or lettuce), or soups.

Go easy on alcohol. Though a drink a day may be good for your heart, alcohol use has been linked to cancers of the mouth, throat, esophagus, liver, colon, and breast. What's more, excess alcohol can contribute to bone thinning, making bones more likely to break if you fall—and can make you wobbly, so falls are more likely.

Strategies to outwit your appetite

Knowing what you should eat and putting such a diet into practice are two different things. Here are some strategies to help control your weight.

Keep a food journal. If you've been gaining weight but aren't sure exactly why, it can be helpful to keep a food journal. Writing down what—and how much—you eat can help you become more aware of habits that are holding you back. One study found that people who recorded what they ate every day lost twice as much weight as people who didn't track their diets. You can do this by hand or with a smartphone app, such as Lose It, MyFitnessPal, MyFoodDiary, MyNetDiary, or SparkPeople.

Weigh yourself frequently. Research reveals that weighing

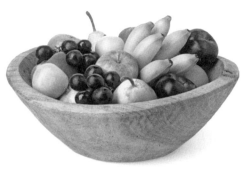

In one study, people who kept a bowl of fruit on the counter weighed 13 pounds less than those who didn't.

yourself doesn't just help you lighten up, it can help you keep pounds off by letting you know if they are starting to sneak back on. You don't need to weigh in every day. While people who monitor their weight daily tend to lose the most weight, weekly weigh-ins are also effective.

Hide snack foods—or better yet, don't buy them. If you keep your salty or sugary snacks on the kitchen counter, find them a new home tucked away in the pantry. If they're not in your line of vision every time you enter the kitchen, you'll be less tempted to eat them. Researchers at Cornell University found that people who stored foods and beverages such as candy, cereal, and soda on their kitchen counters weighed 20 to 26 pounds more than people who kept these items out of sight. Conversely, those who placed a bowl of fruit on the counter weighed 13 pounds less than people who didn't.

Use smaller dishes. Bigger plates, glasses, and bowls almost always lead you to eat too much. The larger the dishes, the more

© hydrangea100 | Getty Images

food you fill them up with—and the more food you load onto your plate, the more you're likely to consume. Simply using a bowl that's 50% larger encourages you to eat 20% more food.

Tame your sweet tooth. Admittedly, this isn't easy. Eating a sugary treat—a candy bar, a cookie, ice cream, a piece of cake—stimulates the reward center in the brain and makes you crave more, so cutting down can be tough. To reduce your sugar consumption, you need to change your brain's expectations of sweetness. Start by substituting fruit for sugary desserts. Fruit delivers a daily dose of sweetness— just less of it. Use sweet spices like cinnamon in cooking. When cravings strike, distract yourself by going for a walk or calling a friend—or try brushing your teeth to deliver the sweet taste of mint.

Eat early in the day. Research increasingly shows that it's better to eat earlier in the day than to pack in the bulk of your calories at night. In part, this has to do with the types of food you're likely to eat as the day advances. Late-night snacks are often the worst. However, metabolic factors may also play a role. A study from Harvard Medical School found that when people ate in the evening, they burned off fewer of the calories than when they ate the identical meal in the morning. Another study found that dieting women who ate lunch after 3 p.m. lost less weight than those

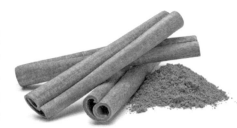

Use sweet spices like cinnamon in cooking to help tame sugar cravings. Herbs like mint can also help satisfy a sweet tooth.

who lunched earlier, even though both groups had similar diets and calorie intakes. Given that food is fuel for your muscles and metabolism, it may be that our bodies are programmed to use calories consumed earlier in the day and store those eaten later.

Fill up with water, soup, and salad before an entrée. Starting meals with low-calorie foods and water can reduce food intake by up to 20%, according to studies.

Get enough sleep. Emerging research reveals that the less you sleep, the more likely you are to put on excess weight. Lack of sleep slows metabolism. The fatigue you feel as a result makes you less likely to exercise. And even more insidious, sleep deprivation changes the balance of hormones governing hunger, making you crave more sweets. Research shows that a lack of sleep can make you eat 300 to 550 more calories a day.

Do you need supplements?

It's best to get nutrients from the foods you eat, not from supplements. That said, taking a daily multivitamin can be a reasonable step for filling gaps in nutrition.

Choose a supplement that gives you the standard recommended daily doses of vitamins and minerals. Avoid those that offer "super" doses of any nutrient. Three specific supplements you might want to ask your doctor about are vitamin D, calcium, and vitamin B_{12}.

- Getting a little extra vitamin D—1,000 to 2,000 IU a day— seems to be good for health. Vitamin D deficiency is very common, especially among older adults and people who don't get much sunlight. Extra vitamin D is good for bone health, because it helps the body absorb calcium from the food you eat.

- The amount of calcium you should get daily rises with age. Men under age 70 and women under age 50 should get 1,000 mg of calcium a day. After that, aim for 1,200 mg a day. Calcium-rich foods include milk and other dairy products and green leafy vegetables. Calcium is often added to cereals, soy milk, breads, and snacks.

- Vitamin B_{12} is another vitamin that can be hard to get from food. It's vital for nerve function, but the body's ability to absorb it from food declines over time. The recommended dietary allowance is 2.4 micrograms per day.

Check with your doctor about which supplements are right for you. He or she can perform simple blood tests to determine whether your levels of vitamin D or vitamin B_{12} are too low. ◆

Maintaining independence

Say you're taking all the right steps to make sure you remain mobile. But does your home—and your larger environment—help or hinder your efforts to maintain your independence? There may be ways you can change things to aid your mobility and prevent injuries. You can also be proactive about planning for a future when your mobility may be limited by age or a chronic health problem.

This report has focused on ways to stay healthy and active so that you have the best possible chances of retaining your mobility and independence. But when something does change—a health problem, or increased frailty with aging—some people feel resistant to making changes in their home, their environment, or their routine. They feel that installing grab bars in the shower or hiring a part-time caregiver is a sign of old age and signals a loss of independence. They keep doing things the same way even if that way is harder and they are putting their own safety at risk.

It's important to keep the bigger goal in mind: preserving your health. If standing in the shower is difficult for you, install a shower seat so you won't fall and break a hip. If you have a health problem that makes shopping at the grocery store painful, have groceries delivered rather than sacrificing a healthy, balanced diet. If you are concerned about driving, maybe there are adaptations you can make (see "Driving: Staying up to the challenge," page 36). Set health as your priority and adapt your environment as needed.

Aging in place

Most people would rather stay in their homes as they grow older instead of moving to a retirement community or nursing home. The CDC defines "aging in place" as "the ability to live in one's own home and community safely, independently, and comfortably, regardless of age, income, or ability level."

Lately there has been a surge of interest in

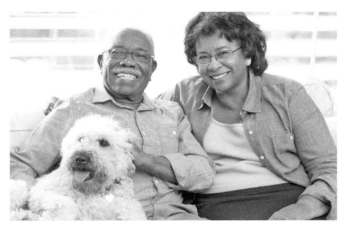

Most people would rather stay in their homes as they grow older than move to a retirement facility. To make that possible, you need to make some adaptations to your home and lifestyle.

research, policies, and design that contribute to the goal of aging in place. Cities are beginning to pay more attention to designing age-friendly streets and public spaces. And a growing number of services are available to help older people modify their homes to make life easier. Technology has also changed what it means to age in place, making it easier to bring goods and services to your door, and offering new ways to monitor and protect your health.

Aging in place isn't about avoiding change. It's about making adaptations to your existing home and lifestyle as you age. Even if you stay in your own home, you should expect to make at least some alterations to accommodate changing physical abilities, as well as modifying some of your routines around the house. Some people are designing and remodeling homes based on universal design principles, which have features that allow a home to accommodate people of varying ages and abilities.

Adapting and fall-proofing your home

Improving your balance, strength, and coordination is a great way to reduce your risk of falls. But tripping hazards at home also pose a risk, so you should periodically make a safety inventory of your home to eliminate fall dangers. Pay special attention to stairs, bathrooms, and the kitchen, which tend to be hot spots for falls.

Over time, you may need to make larger adjustments to your home's design or move to a house that is easier to navigate and maintain. There's a burgeoning industry to help people age in place: the National Association of Home Builders, for instance, now offers a training program for certified aging-in-place specialists who focus on refitting homes for older adults. (A directory of certified specialists can be found at www.nahb.org/CAPSdirectory.) Don't automatically assume you need extensive remodeling; focus modifications on what suits your needs and lifestyle. You can also invest in emergency response systems that give you an added measure of security (see "Technology to keep tabs on you," below).

Throughout the home

- Use flooring that is smooth, nonglare, and slip-resistant. A slippery floor is a fall waiting to happen. Also, carpets and rugs should have a pile that's less than half an inch deep, and rugs should have nonskid pads or backings to keep them from sliding or folding over. Keep floors clear of clutter that someone could trip on.
- Keep hallways well lit, and put night lights in bedrooms, bathrooms, and connecting hallways.
- Keep electrical cords for floor lamps, TVs, phones, and other devices tucked away from where you walk or against the walls.
- Make sure stairs have a handrail that runs the full length of the stairs and just past them, and light switches at the top and bottom. For extra safety, install handrails on both sides of staircases.
- Install a security system that can directly contact police, fire, and emergency medical services.

Technology to keep tabs on you

When you live on your own, safety concerns can arise. The following are just a few of the technologies that make aging in place a safer option.

Sensors. Technologies like Alarm.com's Wellness independent living system (www.alarm.com) use wireless sensors placed throughout your home to monitor your daily activities. The system learns your patterns, like when in the morning you generally go into the kitchen to make coffee, how often you take your medication, and at what time you go to bed. Then it uses algorithms to determine whether you've deviated from your usual routine. For example, if you haven't opened the refrigerator in more than 24 hours, it will send a text message, email, or other alert to the family member(s) you've designated. Because the system uses sensors rather than cameras, it's less invasive to your privacy. You'll pay an upfront cost for installation, plus a monthly subscription fee for the service.

Whole-home monitoring. Wi-fi–enabled security cameras like Nest Cam (https://store.google.com/us/product/nest_cam) and Ring Cam (www.ring.com) let your loved ones see what you're up to on their smartphones and let you check in on your own home when you're away.

Medical alert devices. You've probably seen the commercial with the woman on the floor crying out, "Help! I've fallen and I can't get up." That ad was for Life Alert (www.

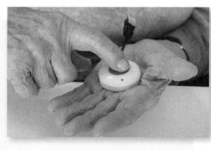

lifealert.com)—one of many medical alert systems that enable you to summon emergency help at the push of a button on a waterproof pendant worn around your wrist or neck. Some companies—like Philips Lifeline (www.lifeline.philips.com)—offer a mobile version that uses GPS to locate you in an emergency.

Pill reminders. People in their 80s take an average of 18 different types of pills per year. Having to juggle so many different medications—each with its own dosing regimen—can lead to mistakes and missed pills. If you rely on your medicines to keep you healthy, these errors could be dangerous. Several products—including E-pill MedTime Station (www.epill.com/epillstation.html) and Med-E-Lert Automatic Pill Dispenser (www.medelert.net)—will help organize your pills and remind you to take them at the right time. Products like MedMinder (www.medminder.com) will also send alerts to your family members, but you'll pay a monthly fee for the service. A lower-tech alternative is PillPack (www.pillpack.com), a full-service mail-order pharmacy that will sort your medications into separate envelopes that tell you when to take them (the envelopes are stamped with both the day of the week and the time of day).

- If you use a wheelchair, make sure the living area, kitchen, and at least one bedroom and bathroom have a five-foot-square clear space to accommodate wheelchair movements. The main bedroom, a full bath, and living areas should be on a single floor, with no stairs separating rooms or areas. Hallways should be at least 36 inches wide, and windows should be low and easy to open, shut, and lock.

House exterior

- For general safety, install lighting at doorways, porches, and walkways. Motion detector lights are best for lighting the way when you come home at night.
- If you live in an area that gets snow, keep supplies like shovels and melting salt handy, and consider paying for a service to clear walkways of snow and ice if it's difficult for you.
- Keep walkways in good repair, with an even surface. Uneven pavement is easy to trip on.
- If you're moving to a new house, choose one with a low-maintenance exterior, such as vinyl or brick.
- Landscape with low-maintenance shrubs and plants.

Entrances and doors

- Make sure you have at least one no-step entrance, lit with a motion sensor light.
- Fix doors to the house so they are easy to unlock and open. If it takes you a while to turn a key, install a keyless entry using a card or remote control. If grip strength is a problem for you, install handles instead of doorknobs. Some companies sell levers that you can attach to a doorknob to serve the same purpose.
- Doors should be at least 32 inches wide—preferably 36 inches.
- Remove any doormats or rugs that you might trip on. Raised thresholds can be lowered or ramps installed, if needed.

Bathroom

- Add grab bars (which are sturdier than towel bars) to your shower or bath. Grab bars are also useful near the toilet for getting up and down. The bathroom is one of the most dangerous rooms of the house and a frequent site of injuries and falls.

- Consider adding a bathing stool or shower seat, along with a handheld shower head attached to a hose. These make it easier to bathe sitting down.
- In the tub, install a nonslip surface, or add a non-slip mat. On the floor, consider using textured tiles, which tend to be less slippery when wet.
- A contrasting border on the edge of the bathroom countertop can make it easier to see.
- Consider making at least one bathroom on the main level wheelchair-maneuverable, with a 60-inch turning radius or acceptable T-turn space, and a clear space that's 36 inches square or 30 inches by 48 inches.

Bedroom

- Rearrange your closet so you can easily reach things you need.
- Take steps to make sure you can get into and out of bed easily and safely. A firm mattress will make it easier, as will a bed that is low enough to the ground that your feet touch the floor when you're sitting on the edge of the bed. Install bedrails to help you raise and lower yourself if needed.
- Put lamps at the bedside that are easy to switch on and off.

Kitchen

- Rearrange cabinets and drawers so you can reach food, dishes, pots, and utensils without straining. Store the heaviest items in places where you don't have to bend down or reach high.
- Keep a sturdy step stool on hand if you have high cabinets that are difficult to reach.
- Install single-lever faucets, which are easier to operate, and counters with rounded corners.

Adapting your lifestyle

In addition to home modifications, you may have to make changes in your lifestyle and routine so that you can remain in your home. Some changes mean paying more for services, but they may be worth the money if they help you avoid an expensive move to an assisted living facility and help you stay in a home you love.

- Ask for help with raking leaves, home repairs, gardening, or snow removal, from either a relative, a neighbor, or a paid service.

- Pay for an occasional housecleaning service to clean areas that are hard for you to reach.
- Hire an in-home companion to help you with household tasks you can't do on your own, such as shopping, cooking, or doing laundry. Sometimes an informal arrangement—such as a college student who lives in a home and provides help in exchange for rent—works well.
- Have groceries or meals delivered. Numerous grocery delivery services—including from major retailers like Amazon, Walmart, Safeway, Stop & Shop, and Whole Foods (now part of Amazon), as well as Instacart—make it easy to keep your pantry stocked. Several services deliver meal kits you can cook yourself. Hot, nutritious meals may also be available through programs like Meals on Wheels America (www.mealsonwheelsamerica.org). Senior centers, community groups, or religious organizations may have similar services.
- Check out transportation options. Some communities offer free or low-cost transportation to medical appointments for seniors or people who are disabled. Other good sources of free or low-cost assistance are religious and community organizations, such as churches or synagogues, councils on aging, and senior centers.
- Make an effort to be in better contact with neighbors and with nearby relatives and friends; try to establish regular check-ins, particularly if you are dealing with health issues.

Finding help

The U.S. Department of Health and Human Services has an Eldercare Locator that connects you to services available in your area, including financial assistance, transportation, long-term care, and volunteer services. See www.eldercare.acl.gov or call 800-677-1116. In addition, the United Way can help you locate resources in your area.

BenefitsCheckUp, a service of the National Council on Aging, connects people 55 or older to benefit programs that cover some costs for rent, property taxes, heating and utility bills, health care, prescription drugs, and other services or goods. You can choose to use the full benefits database or one that focuses only on prescription drug coverage. You can use these free services as often as you like. The questionnaire at www.benefitscheckup.org takes less than half an hour to fill out. It requires personal financial information, but it is confidential. If you appear to qualify for any programs, the service gives you contact information so you can request the benefit. Internet access and computer skills are necessary to fill out the forms.

Assessing your community

The design of a community can affect the mobility of its residents. Although you have limited control over how your neighborhood or city is designed, you can advocate for changes by bringing the issue to your condo or neighborhood association, your city council, or your state representative. Being aware of these issues can also help you decide whether to move, and where. Every neighborhood comes with trade-offs—you may prefer to live close to a family member, for instance, even if it's far from grocery stores. But taking an inventory of how your neighborhood meets your needs can help you find ways to work around the challenges.

Public transportation. Most people outlive their ability to drive. Yet some communities that cater to retirees are far from urban areas with robust public transit systems. And many centers that offer affordable housing and services to older adults are located in suburbs inconvenient to shopping centers and grocery stores. While these places are attractive because they offer quiet, peaceful living "away from it all," they become much more isolating if you can't drive, or if driving is challenging for you. Having access to reliable public transportation could allow you to remain independent and active as you age. Some communities offer special shuttles or dial-a-ride services to seniors and people with disabilities who have trouble getting to transit stops and stations, or who need transport for medical treatment.

Driveability. How easy is it to drive in your community? If you are in an area that's frequently affected by snowstorms, is there a reliable plowing service? Are streets well marked, and can you park easily at grocery stores, medical centers, and other places you frequent?

Walkability. Living in a walkable neighborhood can vastly improve your health and mobility by encouraging you to use your body to get around rather than driving. Even if you regularly go to a gym or work out at home, the ability to easily and safely walk to a grocery store or do other errands on foot will add to your daily activity level. A walkable neighborhood generally has dedicated sidewalks and marked crossings for pedestrians, as well as shops, parks, and other destinations within walking distance. Weather and climate matter too; if you live in a place that is stiflingly hot in the summer or dangerously icy in the winter, that will reduce how much you walk.

Safety. How older adults perceive the safety of their neighborhoods shapes their health. Those who think their neighborhoods are safe are more likely to engage in physical activity outdoors, while those in unsafe neighborhoods are less likely to do so. The resulting decline in physical activity has consequences. One survey of 18,000 people over age 50 found that those who perceived neighborhoods as unsafe were more likely to experience functional decline over a 10-year period and were less likely to recover from mobility problems.

Access to shops and services. Access to grocery stores with fresh food is important for maintaining a healthy lifestyle and also for preserving independence with aging. So is access to pharmacies, clinics, and any other services you depend on for your health.

Access to nature. Does your home have easy access to a park, community garden, lake, or other natural space? These can provide walking destinations and motivate you to get outside and avoid isolation. Research has linked regular access to nature with improvements in health and well-being.

Social environment. Do you have relatives or friends who live near you and whom you visit regularly? Are there places where you can socialize and meet other people, like community centers, fitness centers, or clubs? Are there any neighborhood social activities?

Some people pursue retirement dreams that involve moving to places where they have always wanted to live, only to find they are more isolated from family and friends.

Making a move

Your goal of independent living may be to stay in your own home, but moving to a retirement community with more help and resources available can also help you stay more healthy and active. What's important is that you make a plan based on your own values and priorities, rather than making rushed decisions when a sudden medical setback like a broken hip or stroke makes it necessary. Fortunately, many options are available.

Active adult communities. Also called "55+ communities," these communities either market themselves to adults over 55, or have age restrictions in place so most residents are over 55. They cater to independent adults, so they don't offer assisted living, but many have community activities, like fitness or arts and crafts. In addition to connecting you with like-minded people, these communities provide helpful resources (like lawn care and snow removal), security systems, and opportunities for social interaction.

Senior villages. Beacon Hill Village in Boston, established in 2002, was the first of many formal groups of neighbors helping neighbors with the goal of promoting an active lifestyle, improving health, and reducing isolation among people over the age of 50. The village concept differs from an active adult community in that people age in place, living in their own homes scattered throughout a city rather than in a physically discrete community. Village members pay a fee to hire an expert staff to deliver support services, such as grocery shopping and rides to doctors' visits. They also connect with their neighbors though social and wellness programs, cultural and educational activities, and excursions.

NORCs. A naturally occurring retirement community (NORC) is a neighborhood or housing complex that wasn't planned as a retirement community, but in which a high proportion (usually 40% to 50%) of residents are over 60. The designation enables these communities to receive public or private funding to provide senior-friendly services and coordinated care and support. Your local agency on aging may have information on what is available in your area.

Granny pods. Think of these structures, also called accessory dwelling units, as a more private version of an in-law apartment. A granny pod is a small, prefabricated cottage built in the backyard of one of your adult children. You have privacy, but you can easily visit your children and grandkids—and in case of an emergency, those who care about you are close at hand. Some models include equipment to monitor medical conditions and provide added security (see "Technology to keep tabs on you," page 48).

Continuing care retirement communities. These are similar to active adult communities but have medical staff and facilities on site, so that a person can move from a home to an assisted living unit or nursing bed easily when ill or as his or her needs change. If you move to this kind of community, make sure you are comfortable with the setup of each level of care. These communities often require a high entrance fee as a prepayment for later care, as well as a monthly fee. Make sure the facility has a good track record and is likely to continue to thrive, and that the fee structure makes financial sense for you.

Assisted living. People who can't live on their own because they need help with everyday tasks such as bathing, dressing, making meals, and doing laundry may consider an assisted living facility. This option does not provide round-the-clock nursing care, but many assisted living facilities have nursing homes nearby, so if needs change, residents can transfer to another location. Assisted living can cost around $35,000 to $69,000 per year and is often covered by long-term care insurance, but not private medical insurance or Medicare.

Nursing homes. A nursing home is the most comprehensive level of care for people who are too sick to live alone or to be cared for at home. Some basically look like a hospital, while others are designed to look and feel more like a home. Nursing homes are also the most expensive living situation, costing on average more than $90,000 a year, though facilities differ widely in costs.

Staying social

One measure of successful independence is easy to overlook as you focus on housing, food, and medical care—and that is staying in touch with friends and family. As you retire, you may start to lose your sense of belonging. But social engagements—or even regular phone calls with family and friends—can help you maintain your contacts and feel more engaged with the world. They can keep you on top of current events. And they can just make you happier.

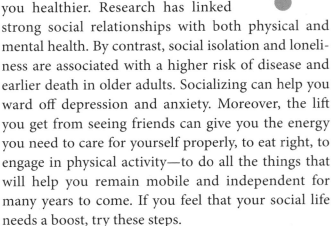

Social connections can also keep you healthier. Research has linked strong social relationships with both physical and mental health. By contrast, social isolation and loneliness are associated with a higher risk of disease and earlier death in older adults. Socializing can help you ward off depression and anxiety. Moreover, the lift you get from seeing friends can give you the energy you need to care for yourself properly, to eat right, to engage in physical activity—to do all the things that will help you remain mobile and independent for many years to come. If you feel that your social life needs a boost, try these steps.

Make a habit. You can strengthen existing relationships by making your interactions more routine. Establishing a weekly call, a regular Sunday brunch, or a monthly outing will keep you from letting your connections lapse.

Find people who share your interests. If you love to read, you could join a book group. If you enjoy cooking, take a cooking class.

Help others. Volunteering with a local charity, religious institution, or nonprofit organization either in person or virtually is a great way to feel connected to others and contribute to your community.

Go online. Facebook and other social media sites make it possible to keep in touch with distant friends and family members, and some research suggests that they may help older adults stay mentally engaged.

Combine physical and social activity. When you take walks, do yoga, or go for a swim with friends, it serves a dual purpose: maintaining your connections while motivating you to move. Both are key to a healthy life moving forward. ▼